AWAY WITH THE CARIES

STUART CRAIG BDS

CONTENTS

"Who would be a dentist?" I've heard some say. Well lots of people actually, which is just as well because like doctors, plumbers, joiners, bus drivers, teachers, nurses, and any job you care to mention…..we all need one at sometime or another.

"How can you spend the whole day looking into peoples' mouths?" Well it was quite easy actually - I used my eyes. Coping with it all was a different matter - it's all in the training.

Why I became a dentist, and not an electrical engineer (which I always fancied), is touched on later, but I am glad I did. It gave me a good career, a purpose in life, a good standard of living, and (here comes the philanthropic bit) a chance to help people and give a sustained contribution to what we refer to as society.

Dentists may fall into the same category as tax inspectors, insurance salesmen and traffic wardens as Joe Public's least favourite people, but hopefully I can address that a little in this book.

What really annoys me is the bad press dentistry tends to get in the media. We've all seen the headlines or leaders: "The pain of the dentist", "The harrowing drill", "The fear and anguish of a dental visit". It is all nonsense, believe me, for I have been on both ends of the drill as, believe it or not, dentists generally have teeth of their own. Routine dental treatment is painless. Sometimes one can be faced with a nasty situation, such as a badly abscessed tooth, or a hyper sensitive nerve, but these can be positively managed without having to scrape the patient off the ceiling.

Television companies love making documentaries or real-life 'fly-on-the-wall' programmes on doctors, midwives, surgeons and vets - and quite rightly too. But have you ever seen one on 'The Dentist'? Whenever some innovation in dentistry is announced the press will invariably begin with the headline:

"The pain at the dentist may soon be a thing of the past."

It was 'a thing of the past' fifty years ago. The vast majority of patients understand that. Sure, some people are anxious about visiting their practice, and that is understandable because dentists do things to you - they treat teeth surgically, not medically, by and large. But most patients have an excellent rapport with their dentist, are on first name terms, respect their opinion and agree with the treatment choices - provided the dentist can communicate well with them.

American dentist Jennifer Gee Schoon-Tong sums up the portrayal of dentists in the media very well. In an online article in 'deardoctor.com' from 2012, she writes:

"Though dentistry is one of the most trusted professions in America, it is seldom portrayed in a positive light in TV, movies, and even social media….I realize (sic) going to the dentist isn't always fun for everyone, or even funny. But it can be.....".

For what it's worth I agree wholeheartedly with her, and love her summing up.

"Right now, a dentist somewhere is relieving someone's pain or giving someone a new smile."

Well said Jennifer.

So this little book is trying to put a smile into dentistry. Hopefully it will achieve that in two ways. Firstly by explaining in simple terms what a dentist actually does in your mouth when you need treatment, and secondly, by sharing a few funny anecdotes that came my way during my 33 years of practice. But before we begin in earnest let me alert the reader to another little game they can indulge in as they flick through these pages. Within the text there are the titles of 28 David Bowie songs. Why? Well he was my rock hero, and I still lament his passing. It's not an original idea, for naturalist and presenter Chris Packham managed to feed about forty Bowie titles into the *Springwatch 2011* live broadcasts. I could have chosen Ed Sheeran, but then I wouldn't have been able to name one!

So – teeth - let's start at the beginning.

What made me want to become a dentist in the first place is covered later on, but I started my career at Glasgow University in 1976, along with about 60 other dental students. The course was five years long and kicked off with intense lectures and labs in chemistry and biology. Next came physiology, biochemistry, pharmacology and anatomy, mixed in with a bit of beer drinking, disco dancing and a fair run of hangovers. By third year we were visiting hospital wards, seeing our own dental patients and studying pathology and the dental sciences. It is fair to say that the course became easier as the years progressed. By the time it was over most of us could crown a tooth with one arm tied behind our back - well maybe not quite, but the expectation of success was upon us.

I loved Glasgow 'Uni' - it is a fine institution and my memories of my time there are mostly happy ones, especially Friday evenings in the Extension Bar of the Union – they were particularly happy.

Our class of budding dentists was a decent bunch, pretty well grounded and keen to have a bit of fun along the way towards blossoming into the health care professionals that the system had designed for us. I quickly made good pals – future colleagues many of whom I still keep in contact with today.

Lectures were intense – there was a lot to learn. I struggled at the chemistry, despite studying it for six years at school, and whizzed through the biology, although I had no knowledge of the subject prior to starting the course and thought a cell was something prisoners were kept in. These were the days before the internet and mobile phones; learning was done by attending lectures and reading. Once in the clinics it was by listening and watching, and not copying the mistakes the chap next to you made.

Anatomy was tough – a bit like learning the Yellow Pages. We spent a lot of time in the dissection room where each group (of students) was allocated the earthly remains of someone who had altruistically given their body, once they were finished with it, to 'medical research'. Ours was an elderly lady whom we named Alice. We were well warned to treat our cadaver with respect, and of course, we did.

Each group consisted of six students and when Alice was uncovered for the first time one of our chaps immediately fainted. This led to a horizontal chain reaction around the room – supine cadavers and supine dental students – where to stick the dissecting scalpel in first? But things soon settled down. Over the years of our studies I think each one of us passed out, not just in the graduating sense but in the loss of consciousness sense I mean. If not exactly swooning onto the floor most of us, at some point, gave a mumbled excuse and left the room. One girl fainted on seeing her first tooth being extracted, another on looking at some exceedingly fresh post-mortem specimens. Poor Alex passed out in the Oral Medicine clinic, but he had a decent excuse – his best pal was taking 20ml of blood out of a vein in his arm at the time. Well, we all had to learn how to perform venesection! As for me, I had to leave a theatre at Canniesburn Hospital where I was 'assisting' - more likely impeding - a surgeon as he removed a benign tumour from an old chap's upper lip. The surgeon inadvertently cut through a small artery and I got showered in the red stuff. It was in my eyes, on my face and in my hair – which at that time resembled a curly ball of wool (think Leo Sayer or Robert Powell and I think you'll get the picture). Two minutes later I was in the back room with my head between my knees. I recovered quickly, however, and was soon back in, impeding again. Generally it is worse watching a surgical procedure than it is actually doing it. I never particularly liked watching a dental surgeon digging out a broken down molar, but when it came to doing it myself then I was fine. In fact it could be good fun.

My hair had been the focus of attention sometime before this episode. In second year I was working with my lab partner in a biochemistry lab in the Boyd Orr Building when, on leaning a touch too far over the Bunsen burner I set my curls alight. I never noticed, but my colleague suddenly stared at me aghast, then threw a beaker of water over me.

"What the f...! What in the world are you doing? What's that smell?"

"Your hair's on fire!"

I was unhurt, thanks to his quick reactions, but the lab stank of burnt Afro for days afterwards. Students would arrive at the lab, screw up their noses and say "what's that awful smell?"

"Oh it's okay, Stuart just set his hair alight."

A nervous look in a mirror revealed my worst fears – my hair now looked as though it belonged to Arthur Scargill. I had to hide under a cap and sneak off to the hairdressers.

Back to anatomy, and a lot of our year failed their first sitting of the anatomy degree exam, I didn't – I say smugly, as I had spent a whole Easter with an anatomy book glued to my face and guessing portentously a couple of questions that would come up in the exam. These questions would go something like: 'describe the course of the glossopharyngeal nerve'. This is like someone asking you to recall in great accuracy the route of the M6 from Wigan to Carlisle. Which roads branch off it? What bridges cross it? Where is the A49 in relation to it? What are the names of the service stations along its route and how much is a bacon roll in each one?

In lectures there was always some wag that was waiting to pounce on the slightest gaff or hesitation by the lecturer. In an anatomy lecture Dr Young was settling us down prior to enlightening us on the gastro-intestinal system.

"Today we're going to do the whole of the alimentary system."

"What about the rest of it?" Charlie shouted out, quick as a fart.

One of the funniest was actually at a postgraduate course, many years later, that I attended at the Royal College of Surgeons and Physicians in Glasgow. The subject was radiography. Our lecturer was the very proper Dr Primm. Her audience that evening was a clutch of around forty dentists and she was discussing the potential risks of everyday objects and appliances to our wellbeing. As an example she reminded us that digital alarm clocks gave off tiny amounts of radioactivity.

"Well I have such a clock on my bedside cabinet, so when I discovered that it emitted harmful rays I moved it further away from me," she continued, but without anticipating her audience's reaction to her next line added "well, when it's every night a few inches matter."

This brought the house down. It took five minutes to restore order, whereupon a red-faced Dr Primm stuttered, "I don't *do* jokes like that!" Neither she does.

By the end of the third year of our course we were exclusively captives of the dental hospital, although we were sometimes let home in the evenings. At this fine, but somewhat scary establishment, we entertained the clinicians, and they entertained us. I have very fond memories of my time there. In the Child Dental Health clinic I have particularly fond memories - for I met my future wife there, our eyes meeting over an extraction. It was the clinicians there who particularly entertained us. I remember experienced dentist Mr Gould trying to calm a screaming child who clearly wanted to be elsewhere. Alarmed at the effect this was having on the waiting room he left the clinic to address the waiting hoards.

"Look, I'm only washing my hands - I haven't even touched him yet!" It was the same clinician who, on filling a child's baby tooth, reassured the lad by explaining that he was "just putting worms and sausages in his tooth."

With few exceptions I found the relationship between student and clinician an excellent, professional one. Our teachers were clearly doing their best to get us to qualify - well it would get us off their hands.

Students often get a bad name but looking around me as the five years progressed I was quietly proud to see a steady professional attitude seep through the adolescent fuzz of our student minds as we were gradually processed by our tutors into becoming fine, upstanding dentists, even though we did most treatments sitting down. However there was the odd occasion when one of us, or some of us, let our guard down.

Each 'year group' of dental students at Glasgow gave themselves a name and over the five years held charitable events to help raise funds that would eventually pay for our Final Year Dinner, while at the same time raising cash for worthwhile causes, such as the homeless, the starving and replacing the front left wing of the year captain's Ford Fiesta. Our year group was called *Amylase Masticator* (amylase being an enzyme, but the designation suggesting someone who can't be bothered chewing their food – like King Edward VII, apparently). We held dances, jumble sales, car treasure hunts (that was when the Fiesta got bashed) and various honourable happenings. In June 1978 some smart person thought that it would be a good idea to head for Millport, have a charity cycle twice around the island, and then maybe go to the pub.

We set off for Great Cumbrae - Millport as it is referred to by your average Glaswegian – on a gloriously sunny Saturday. The first part went well enough, the cycling that is, but back at the George Hotel in Millport things got a little bit out of hand. Davie managed to use his bottom to push a beer glass through the window and onto the street, twenty feet below. Fortunately nobody was standing underneath, apart from the local bobby. This led to a couple of our number being sheepishly escorted to the ferry with a dire warning never to set foot on the Island of Great Cumbrae again or else they'd be banished to Little Cumbrae Island.

Back in the professional confines of the dental hospital our lecturers and clinicians were doing their best to get us through the written and practical exams. Being examined on a particular treatment for a patient was scary, nerve jangling stuff – for the student's nerves, I mean, the patients were usually numbed. We had to perform several fillings for part of our final exams. Each stage of the process, from diagnosis to tooth preparation to restoration of the tooth, was inspected and graded. With some fillings a special metal band (called a matrix band) had to be placed around the tooth so that the filling could be formed to the correct shape and would then contact the adjacent tooth properly (an important issue). On the morning of my exam, I discovered to my terror that the Dean of the dental school was the examiner. Yes, the boss, the professor himself. So, head down, I set to work and prepared the tooth. The cavity I had prepared got an approving nod from him and I then applied the matrix band – not without considerable fiddling. This also had to be checked, so he came over to inspect.

"Mmm. Very unconventional."

"Really?" I stuttered.

"Yes, you've put the band on upside down, but that will still do the job. Very unconventional."

He passed me, and I forever held him in great awe for his decency.

Clinicians were only human too, you'll be glad to hear. One day in the surgical clinics we were being shown how to give an 'inferior dental block'. An inferior dental block is not a subordinate, stupid student, but an injection given with a long needle very specifically behind the last lower tooth to *block* the nerve which supplies sensation to all the lower teeth on that side.

It is used routinely by dentists as it is a very effective way of numbing all these teeth in one go. But it has to be given carefully: too far forwards and it won't work, too far back and there is a risk of anaesthetising the *facial nerve* which is a motor (rather than sensory) nerve that makes the muscles on one side of your face work. Numbing the facial nerve inadvertently is not dangerous, but the patient needs eye protection until the anaesthetic wears off, as he or she will not be able to blink for four hours. This was all being explained to our small group by Dr Smyth-Robertson, who then called on a volunteer to be 'blocked'. It wasn't me, I was hiding at the back of the room, along with the rest of the guys. Jennifer stepped forward, and we received another lecture from Dr Smyth-Robertson about which intra-oral landmarks to look for to avoid numbing the wrong nerve. He gave her a block and we waited. Five minutes passed and he asked Jennifer if her lower lip was now numb on one side – a telling indication of successful anaesthesia. She replied no, in a rubbery, slurred voice. There she was, the right hand side of her face paralysed, from eyebrow to chin. Dr Smyth-Robertson was apologetic, we all grinned from ear to ear. Jennifer could only grin on one side, had she felt like it.

Half way through final year I earned my first penny as a dental worker. I was filling some poor chap's tooth in the clinic when one of my colleagues approached me, red faced and clearly stressed. He had been similarly trying to fill a molar in a fellow student a few chairs away from me.

"Stuart, I've been trying to fill this tooth for the last hour, but the amalgam keeps falling out. The prof is doing the rounds and he's heading back my way soon to check if I've finished. I'll give you a fiver if you can get the filling to stay in."

This was an offer I couldn't resist, so I ambled over, did a bit more cavity preparation with the drill and filled the cavity with silver amalgam. It seemed to work, well it worked long enough for the prof to pass it. I got my fiver.

Soon the Final exams arrived and I was feeling quite confident. We now had a new Dean, whom I didn't know very well. We only ever had one conversation, which was held in the lift. I was already in it, heading for the top floor of the Dental Hospital when he entered it on level two. Just the two of us. He looked at me and gave the slightest nod.

"Good morning sir." I bravely muttered, feeling that I should show at least a modicum of sycophancy, in case he should be examining my practical exam the following week.

"Good morning Mr Craig," he replied as the doors opened and he prepared to disappear down the corridor of the fifth floor, "and I hope you'll be getting your haircut before the exams." He looked back at me and added "and get rid of those bangles." I was amazed he knew my name.

The two silver bangles that had sat on my left wrist for five years were there in homage to my idol David Bowie. To this day I wear my watch on my right wrist, because the bangles were on my left. Well I recognise good advice when I hear it. To hell with fashion; the next day they were gone, for good, and so was most of my hair – although until recently it has tried to grow back in again.

I passed the Finals and couldn't believe my luck: I was a dentist. I vowed I would never sit another exam again, and never have.

When I graduated from Glasgow University I started work as a dental associate in Lanarkshire, where I remained for over six years. A *dental associate* treats patients within a practice under a high level of clinical freedom. The monies earned by the associate, both NHS and private, are totalled up each month and a percentage is given to the associate – usually between 40-50%. This is actually a good arrangement both for the associate and the practice owner (principal). The principal is receiving a good return from the associate, but the associate has no other expenses – materials, staff wages, rent and lots of other fixed costs are all paid by the principal. So there can be good dollar days for both parties. Fees to the dental technician (for making dentures and crowns) are paid by the associate, as is the mid-morning roll and sausage.

My position in Lanarkshire was a great job, and I was surrounded by caring dentists and nurses, who did their best to support me in my early years. I was so green and looked like I had just stepped out of my school shorts. A patient asked the receptionist one day if I was on the *Job Creation Scheme*. One of the dentists at the practice thought this was hilarious and would tell it to every second patient who came in.

It was enlightening and educating to have left the dental hospital environment behind and be part of a busy family practice; to see the application of dentistry in a thriving community. The quality of work from the dental partners I worked with was very high and set a standard I aspired to. It was hard work, of course, and treatments didn't always head in the direction they were supposed to; neither did I. I worked at two different practices, a few miles apart. I drove to work from Glasgow each morning, travelling to each practice on alternate days. On two occasions I turned up at practice number one, only to realise I was supposed to be at practice number two.

Eventually many dentists have the ambition to own their own practice, so in 1984 I started planning my independent future and three years later bought a shop in Glasgow and converted it to a small dental surgery. This cost me every penny I had, and with four children now on the scene it was a difficult time – though looking back, a great adventure. Until the surgery got up and running I worked part time in a rather seedy area, which shall remain anonymous. The patients were fine - apart from the scary ones – and I spent considerable time trying to sort out the dental problems of some folk who evidently wanted to be somewhere else, pharmacologically speaking. It was heading back to the car in the dark November evenings after a busy session that were intimidating, and it wasn't helped when the practice principal told me that the streets were more dangerous than the charmingly menacing village Midsomer. I didn't last long there as soon my little practice was functional. I loved the thrill of running my own dental practice. Everything was fine except I didn't have enough patients, so within three years I found myself in partnership with my soon-to-be long-standing colleague. We now jointly-owned a family practice in Glasgow's south-side, and we were busy busy busy.

The NHS offers dentists good rewards, but they have to work hard to get them, and they work within the numerous, and ever-growing, constraints of the National Health Service. The system in England for remunerating dentists changed some years ago, but in Scotland we hung on to the 'item-of service' system. Basically, in Scotland, dentists receive a fee for each item of treatment that they do. Each treatment option has a fee attached to it, and the dentist is obliged to charge the patient their share of that fee, currently 80%. This does not apply if the patient is on benefits, is under 18 or pregnant, or all three.

In my opinion, which is all you are getting here, this is a fair system, as patients only pay for the treatment they get, not what they *might* need. Dental examinations are free, fortunately. It is imperative that anyone can seek free advice from their dental health professional, rather than nip across the road to bother their GP.

There were days when I would see 50 patients a day, over a shift that ran from 0830 to 1800. I remember reading an article fairly recently from a polish dentist who had come over to Scotland to work. He stated that work was difficult in Poland because sometimes he had to see 35 patients a day! Welcome to Scotland – which of course you are.

However, being a dental practitioner is a very rewarding and fulfilling vocation, and as you shall see on later pages, there were some smashing people to meet and some fun to be had. Sometimes, while filling a tooth or preparing one for a crown I would look down at my gloved hands and think 'my goodness, how did I get here?' It was a privilege to work on your fellow human kind, trying – and usually succeeding – in putting right whatever dental problem they had. I never lost sight of that and forever felt humbled by the trust that others put in me and my training.

But enough of the soppy stuff, let's look at what dentists actually do.

FILL IT UP, PLEASE

So what does a dentist *do* at a check-up? And what are those tools he or she is holding? Well it is incumbent on a dentist to check the teeth and the soft tissues thoroughly. To aid this, we use a mouth mirror, and a pointed probe. The mirror allows the dentist to look at upper teeth and awkward hidden corners of the mouth without having to stand on his head. The mirror also pushes back lips and tongue to obtain better vision, and can also be used to reflect light into dark corners to obtain a better view. It also makes a handy shield, protecting soft tissues against the whims of fast drills and sharp instruments. Some rotary, polishing discs can jam between teeth, when they then become wheels and try to treat your cheek as the outside lane of the M6.

Teeth are checked for mobility, for decay (caries) and for damage. Their relationship with their neighbours is examined and any adjustment or treatment required is duly noted. Gums are examined to determine their health. Fillings are probed to make sure they are sound and don't need replaced or repaired. The bite (occlusion) is checked and the soft tissues are examined to make sure they are healthy. You can be assured that the dentist has also taken into account the patient's general well-being too. All this can be done fairly quickly and effectively in a systematic manner – thus leaving plenty of time to chat about the football or what was on the telly last night. For although some people are nervous about a visit to the dentist – and we will discuss that in more detail further on – for many their routine check-up is very much a social event too.

The dentist clearly has to write up detailed notes on the findings, or lack of them, at a check-up, and all actual treatments need noted in detail; I won't bore you with dental charting or the hieroglyphics we use. A treatment plan is formed and written down, or more likely entered onto the patient's computer records. For the majority of my career paper notes were taken, but now computer software companies have designed a constellation of colour-coded icons which the dentist or nurse click to produce a screen-full of treatment items. Patients' notes are, of course, confidential, and you can rest assured that the names I assign to the various patients mentioned in this book are fictitious.

Non-clinical, personal notes can be added to the notes. I often noted what the patient did for a living, where they were next going on holiday and anything unusual or interesting that they might have muttered through frozen lips. It took them by surprise at their next visit when I asked them how Torremolinos was. Names of pets, a change in their job, who their new wife was (careful with that one), their favourite malt could all be noted. Sometimes looking back a few pages in a patient's records I would dig up some historical fact they hadn't realised I'd scribbled down.

"I take it Thumper the rabbit has passed away by now?"

"Did you ever marry Miss Scarlet? Oh it was Ms Blue!" Endearing stuff like that.

Cryptic notes were sometimes written too, and I'm not going into that – it would be giving away too many secrets, like David Copperfield telling you how he makes a bus disappear in front of your eyes.

So a treatment plan has been concocted, and dutifully explained to the patient. Often no treatment is required, especially with regular patients who look after their mouths, but if there are corrections that should be made, then it is really the dentist's duty to carry out treatment, as long as the patient understands what is proposed and is willing: they have to give consent.

Some patients were intrigued by the fine detail of their treatment plan, others would have nodded tacitly if I had suggested taking out all their upper teeth and sticking in someone else's. I preferred the former type of patient, who was interested in their mouth and wanted to know exactly what you intended to do. All implications, positive or otherwise, have to be explained and then time allocated to carry out the treatment.

Some dentists like to carry out as much treatment as possible at that first appointment, but unless it was something simple, I preferred to give further appointments, so that both dentist and patient knew what was up next, at future visits.

One of the commonest treatments is having a filling done, or repaired. So what is a filling – apart from the inside of a sandwich? Fillings have been placed in holes in teeth for about two centuries now. To put it simply, a tooth can become decayed, causing a hole to appear. Without intervention the decay will progress, destroy more tooth tissue and creep surreptitiously towards the nerve, deep inside the tooth. If the nerve becomes irritated then so does the patient: pain, infection...you know the story. In order to prevent further damage to the tooth, the dentist removes the decay and fills the hole. That is a filling. It is designed to repair the damage and prevent further problems.

Filling materials have to remain soft (plastic) until the dentist is finished packing it into the cavity, and then need to set quickly. Generally the material is either a metal amalgam alloy or a white composite material. Once mixed, amalgam sets in about ten minutes, composite materials set in about five seconds when a strong light is shone on them by the dentist. Both these materials have their advantages and disadvantages, as you would expect. Amalgams have been around since the early 1800s and are delivered to the tooth as a powder/liquid mix. The powder is an alloy of silver and tin, and often copper and zinc. The liquid is elemental mercury. And herein lies the potential problem. Mercury is toxic in its elemental (liquid) form as the body has a bit of trouble excreting it. However, when it is placed in the tooth as a filling it has been mixed thoroughly with the powdered alloy and is rendered safe. The mixing is done in a sealed machine. Some folk may tell you that amalgam is not safe and will cause all sorts of diseases from piles to scrofula. Personally, I believe it is perfectly safe and a wonderful material to fill teeth as it satisfies a lot of physical properties required of a filling. The main problem with it is that it does not bond to tooth enamel, and it is silvery-grey.

Composites are tooth-coloured and are used on front teeth and back teeth. They are light-cured (the dentist or nurse shines a blue light of specific wavelength on them to make them 'set') and can bond very well to tooth enamel. A special resin is painted onto the tooth prior to curing, which helps the bond.

Gold has also been used to fill teeth, but less commonly now. Again, the main problem with gold fillings is the colour, and the cost, but it is a very durable material and was once very popular.

I could write a whole book on filling materials but will spare you here. The best person to ask about which fillings are suitable in which situation is your own dentist.

This brings us to the problem in the first place. Why does a tooth decay? Well up until the 18th century it was thought to be caused by worms. In those days the chap that pulled out your tooth was the same guy who shoed your horse. Can you imagine the scenario when you visit the blacksmith in pain.

"I'm sorry Mr Smith, your tooth is full of worms and will have to come out. I can fit your mule with a nice pair of metal shoes too, for a couple of extra groats."

Over the years the dental practitioner evolved from the blacksmith to the barber.

"A short back-and-sides please, oh and could you remove that troublesome molar top left while you're at it."

So what really causes tooth decay? Think of it like this: your mouth contains all kinds of bacteria – billions of them. Some are nice, friendly ones and some are potentially nasty. Some of the nasty ones like to eat sugar – the sugar that's left lying around when you munch on a chocolate bar or sticky bun. These bugs eat the sugar and pee out acid as a waste product. This acid dissolves tooth enamel, creates a hole, allows more bacteria to get deep inside the tooth, and creates an even bigger hole. When this hole gets near the pulp (nerve) of a tooth it can irritate it causing pain. If unchecked the nerve tissue will die and become infected. The patient has thus gone from savouring a sticky bun to having a dental abscess. It doesn't happen overnight, but I can assure you it happens.

How do you stop this hideous sequence of affairs? Eat less sugar, brush your teeth with a fluoride toothpaste and visit your dentist frequently for check-ups. By examining your teeth a dentist can very accurately spot early decay, either by using his eyes or by taking a radiograph (X-ray). Once spotted he or she can fix it, usually by filling the tooth. Remember, fillings don't just restore the hole, they also help to prevent further deterioration. This is why the dentist uses drills and scraping instruments to gain access to the cavity and prepare it in such a way that whatever it is filled with it *stays* filled with. Amalgam fillings are often dove-tailed into the cavity, composites are bonded into it.

Drills get a bad name – they shouldn't, they are extremely efficient little gadgets. The cavity has to be 'prepared' in order to clean out the decay, remove any bits of unsupported tooth that are left and to contour the cavity to the desired shape, commensurate with the filling staying in. There are two types of drill – fast and slow. In both cases the actual cutting tool is called a *bur*, and the holder is the *handpiece*. Burs for the *fast drill* are made from diamond, tungsten carbide or steel. Burs for the *slow speed* are usually steel. The *fast drill* is….well, very fast! Its whole purpose in life is to cut through enamel and fillings very quickly and to achieve this it is powered by compressed air, thus the *whoosh*y noise it makes. The bur at the business end also has to be water cooled - as it is rotating at around 400,000 revs per minute - otherwise the tooth being drilled will overheat and the nerve tissue within will be roasted – like an oven chicken.

The *slow speed* drill is, by definition, much slower and gives the dentist a greater tactile sense of what he or she is drilling through. It is used to remove decay delicately. There is no water spray with this, and no *whoosh*, but there is more vibration. All types of burs and rotary devices can be attached to this kind of drill, which makes it a very versatile instrument – it's great for polishing the wife's jewellery.

So drills should not get a bad name as they perform their task exceedingly well, painlessly if local anaesthetic is used judiciously and, this is the important bit, quickly. Be reassured that all burs and handpieces are thoroughly cleaned and then sterilised between patients.

People love talking about dentists' drills, don't they? These useful instruments have attained a notoriety just one step down from the Spanish Inquisition. I bet the SI would have loved to have had them in their torture toolkit. One Saturday my colleague was unblocking a street drain right outside our Glasgow practice using his Kango 1900/KW50 super XL200. Some clever road worker had cemented the pavement outside the surgery window and covered the drain. As he worked away he spotted a patient walking up the street towards him, and he realised that a joke about a drill was forthcoming.

"Oh good morning, sir, I see you're using a different kind of drill this morning."

"Not at all, Mr Pry, it's the same one! See you on Monday morning."

Decay, or 'caries' to give it the proper medical name, can be looked upon as being a bit like dry rot in the timbers of your hall. This can spread insidiously and silently, without grief, for a while. But eventually it needs to be thoroughly removed, the surrounding wood treated and then in-filled. Decay similarly needs proper removal and the cavity treated with nerve-friendly cements to protect it and then filled. Teeth can actually repair themselves, deep down, by laying down new dentine tissue to protect the nerve. To encourage this natural healing process cements rich in calcium hydroxide are used to cover the deep layer of the cavity and to provide an insulating barrier against thermal changes passing down through the filling, such as when hot tea is sipped or cold lager imbibed.

Older patients would tell me that they would never have a local anaesthetic to 'freeze the teeth' when having fillings done – and sometimes when having teeth removed (extracted)! Nowadays a local anaesthetic will be offered, if appropriate. Anaesthetics are discussed in a later chapter, but can be divided into general or local. A general anaesthetic knocks you out cold and has little place in dentistry nowadays. A 'local' will be familiar to most reading this, and are very effective and safe drugs. Mostly they are based on a derivative of cocaine, and numb nerves without inducing the euphoric bit – otherwise there would be queues outside every dental practice in the land!

Having a tooth prepared, or drilled, for a filling or crown isn't necessary painful without a local anaesthetic, but in most people it will be very sensitive. Some folk do not have very sensitive teeth and will let you know they do not need or want a local. That's fine – they know their own mouths. Most patients will have no idea of the extent of work the dentist wants to do and so will want a local. These people are wise! Nobody would drill into one of my teeth without a local. The outer covering of a tooth is enamel, which is very highly calcified and contains no nerve fibres. Beyond enamel, just 2mm further down, is dentine, and in most people this is sensitive to disturbance by dentists, and other stimuli. In many people there is a gap in the enamel, at the neck of the tooth, where it enters the gum, leaving exposed dentine: this is a very common cause of sensitivity.

To make the drilling procedure comfortable, and to prevent the dentist having to chase the patient around the chair - or the room – a local is given gently into the gum above the tooth to be prepared. I normally warmed the glass cartridges of local anaesthetic to render the solution close to blood temperature and thus more comfortable to inject. By injecting slowly dental injections can be as near painless as possible -I have given injections without the patient realising it. The solution will permeate through the gum and bone towards the end of the root of the tooth, where the supplying nerve is to be found. Within a few minutes the tooth can be drilled painlessly. Local can also be injected into a spot where a bigger nerve is located, and thus numb a whole region of the mouth. This is called a block, as described earlier.

The same drugs and injection techniques are deployed for taking a tooth out. In fact, sometimes less local is needed for an extraction as there is no requirement for the nerve of the doomed tooth to be numbed, merely the tissues around it. Dentists sometimes place a 'topical' anaesthetic onto the injection site before giving the local. This is a cream or gel that numbs any small area of gum that the needle comes into contact with. This can render the administration of a local painless, which is particular useful when treating young children, or other dentists, or the patient that brings you a cake each time she attends.

Block injections have a very profound effect and it is wise to warn the patient not to bite their numbed lips afterwards. This may sound unnecessary but patients love to play with a numb lip, especially if it is their own. The disassociation and lack of sensation makes the lip feel like rubber. First they start by pulling it through their teeth. This advances to a little nibble, and then a wee chew. Oblivious to the blood now running down their chin they pretend their lip is a lump of fillet steak. When the anaesthetic wears off, four hours later, they have a hole in their lower lip and a fleshy bit hanging off it. And it is the dentists' fault! Well actually it is if the dentist never warned them. This masochistic behaviour is not confined to children, I've seen a few adults go through the same mutilation, despite being warned. Fortunately lips heal quickly and thoroughly.

As well as numbing the teeth, and as a consequence the adjacent lip, the tongue will also sometimes be affected. It is perhaps less cerebrally rewarding to chew the tongue but, again, if not warned, there are those out there who will find a way to do it. The result will be sorer!

There are many dental treatments that will not require a local anaesthetic - your dentist knows best what these are. For example, drilling into a root-treated tooth, trimming small areas of enamel and, of course, denture work. Cutting a large hole in the live tooth of someone who is a pain-in-the-arse could also be included in this list, but never was. I can recall an unusual exception to one of those, however. A patient had been fitted with a new denture, following extractions, and despite being told to return to the surgery the next day if the denture was digging into their gum he decided to wait to see if things settled down. They didn't, and when he turned up at the practice a week later he had an ulcer under his upper lip so large, deep and painful that I had to give him a local anaesthetic just to get his denture out. I gave him a bit of a row.

Dentists spend a lot of their undergraduate time learning how to make fillings, so they tend to be pretty good at it by the time they are released on the general public. So the next time your dentist tells you that there is a bit of dry rot on your upper first molar don't be unduly alarmed – it can usually be fixed.

Teeth may need filled for reasons other than caries. The tooth may have fractured due to a trauma. The most commonly seen trauma that a dentist has to deal with is when a small child runs into a chair, or another small child's head, or propels himself over the handlebars of his new bike – yes it's usually boys who engage in this type of behaviour. If the child is under, say, six or seven, and only has baby (deciduous) teeth then there is not much that needs to be done, apart from reassurance. There may be much blood, and lots of tears (usually from the parent), and maybe the teeth have been pushed out, or back, or into the gum, or completely knocked out. But it is of no great consequence for the mouth will heal quickly and the teeth may recover their position over a short time – unless they're lying in the school playground. The second (permanent) teeth are not likely to be affected.

When the child is older, trauma can be more devastating. Commonly upper front incisors are the victim. In the young upper jaw these new teeth can look huge, and they are vulnerable. After a knock they can be chipped, but can also be nudged into a position they are not used to being in, or knocked out completely. I will broach the subject of 'knocked -out' teeth in the next chapter. If the teeth are now in the wrong place they can usually be put back in line, but may need subsequent root-treatment. If chipped they can be filled with composite. Often the fracture line is a diagonal across the face of the tooth, sometimes the nerve tissue (pulp) is exposed – in which case the nerve will have to be removed and the tooth root-treated. Again, I will cover root-treatments later on.

A very common cause of trauma, to a front incisor, in a young adult is being hit in the mouth by a bottle of beer. I don't mean an act of unforgivable violence; usually the victim is holding the bottle. They are standing at the bar, about to take another sip, when someone inadvertently nudges them in the back. The bottle hits off an upper central incisor and *crack*! I have seen this so many times. Use a glass!

It is an upsetting event for child and parent when a dental trauma occurs, so both parties need to be reassured and the child dealt with in a sympathetic manner. I remember one wee lad of about seven arriving with his mum in a fluster of minor panic one afternoon. He had lost his upper baby incisor in an accident in the school playground. His school uniform was splattered with blood and his face streaked with tears. Once on the chair he calmed down quickly, although mum looked as though she needed a gin and tonic. I asked him gently what had happened, realising that he would need no active treatment, just a bit of TLC.

"It was play -time and I was running after my pal. A big boy ran across me and I ran into him," he sniffled articulately.

"That's a shame," I said in my kindly voice, "and you knocked your tooth out, and there's a bit of blood, but you'll be fine. Tell me, what state was the big boy in?"

The lad thought for a few seconds and replied, "he was tall, long trousers, brown hair, a white shirt, he had a tie......."

Even the mum drew a smile at that one, so we put the gin and tonic back in the cupboard.

A significant part of the average dentists' week is spent repairing broken teeth. Usually the tooth has already been filled and a corner of it (cusp) has fractured off. It always amazed me why patients with a mouth full of heavy fillings would continue to chew toffees and other sticky foods, causing repeated fractures and frequent visits to the surgery. Very often the patient considered the damage unrepairable, and it was nice to reassure them that their latest bit of frenzied destruction could be fixed, and usually fairly quickly. It would be fair to say that I would spend a fair bit of every January fixing broken cusps that had fractured on the Christmas *Quality Street*. By February the supply of caramels had usually dried up. Some patients' ability to persistently devastate their fillings and teeth was astounding. Their mouths were like the Forth Bridge – constantly needing attention.

"That's you sorted again, Mrs Marzipan, see you again next week."

Very rarely a tooth would break on a foreign object in food. I had a lady who badly fractured a molar on a stone which was hiding in a bag of frozen peas. Another broke a porcelain crown on a nut; I don't mean a Brazil nut or almond, I mean a stainless steel one. My dear wife, Clare, contrived to split an upper premolar right down the centre longitudinally on an olive stone while on holiday in Spain. On our return I then had to open the surgery specially for her on Easter Sunday so that I could extract it – the tooth, not the olive stone.

Teeth may need restored for reasons other than decay or fracture. There is a triumvirate of tooth-loss known as 'attrition, abrasion and erosion' which dentists increasingly spend their time trying to address. Attrition is where tooth enamel, and ultimately dentine, wears down due to the teeth grinding together. For some folk grinding their nashers has become their favourite pastime, but have sympathy, for they often grind while asleep. The subsequent tooth loss (and I mean the loss of tooth substance here, not the loss of a number of teeth) can become extreme and lead to sensitivity, pain in the jaw joints, poor appearance and divorce; the latter due to the noise they make nocturnally while having a decent grind. The problem for the dentist is restoring the lost tooth tissue, for simply filling over the damaged areas is not an option – the patients will grind through the fillings in days.

One note of reassurance here: young children often grind their baby teeth, but with no ill effects, it's when the child reaches 40 that it becomes a problem, as by then teeth can sometimes be worn right through to the nerve.

Abrasion is different, but refers to a similar tooth-loss process where an outside agent has ground away the enamel – usually over- zealous tooth brushing. This can leave notches etched into the neck of the tooth and is usually due to using the brush in the wrong direction: not 'up and down' as we were all taught, but 'side-to-side'.If a toothbrush is used with too much force along a horizontal plane then the resulting damage can resemble the notch a wood cutter achieves on a tree truck when felling it. Abrasion is more easily treated as there are wonderfully adhesive filling materials that can plug the gaps.

Erosion is arguably the worst of the three as this is much commoner in younger people. It is a term used to describe chemical dissolution of tooth enamel, usually from carbonic acid in fizzy drinks. In my opinion as little as a can of these demon drinks daily can cause a general loss of enamel, and then dentine, over the whole tooth surface. This leads to a loss of architecture of the tooth, producing sensitivity and a real headache when it comes to restoring the damage. Best advice is to avoid fizzy drinks, even sugar-free ones as it is the acidity of the bubbly stuff in them that causes the problem. I have seen many ten year olds with significant erosion that will be very difficult to treat without the use of multiple crowns.

Most folk are generally very good at describing their symptoms if they are having bother; but then dentists should be pretty good at listening out for the tell-tale signs that aid their diagnoses. Phrases like: it is sore when I bite down on it, it is sensitive when I eat ice cream, the pain goes up to my ear, all help the dentist come to an appropriate conclusion.

I read years ago that a gorilla in an American zoo had learned to communicate that it was suffering from toothache. The clever ape could 'deaf sign' for pain, could point to where in its mouth it was feeling it and could even grade the pain on a 1-10 scale. Two offending teeth were extracted. How clever. I've met some humans who would have struggled communicating that.

One of the danger signs, for the dentist, was when a patient sat on the chair and then produced a shopping list of complaints. I always encouraged patients to write down their symptoms if they thought they might forget something when sitting in the dental chair or on the doctor's couch. But when the list was written on a length of till-roll then I knew I was in for an extended session. As they reached the end of their list I was often tempted to say "…..and two dead pigeons in the cold water tank!" I think I did actually say this once, during a lapse in concentration, but either the lady didn't hear me (deafness was on her list as well) or she had never seen *Fawlty Towers*.

How does an appointment system work? Well sometimes it just doesn't. I tried to stick rigidly to mine, while my colleague often treated it as a rough guide to how his day was panning out.

Basically, a patient would phone or call in to make an appointment, and an appropriate amount of time would be allocated, and their name entered into the appointment book, or latterly the computer. Some time was left open for the inevitable emergencies that would appear. *Real* emergencies, that would be seen as soon as possible, included: pain, bleeding from a socket following an extraction, painful swelling, sores from newly fitted dentures, sharp edges rubbing against the tongue, young children with sudden problems. Other less urgent problems would be fitted in where there was appropriate time to fix them. On bad days there could be a dozen emergencies all needing attention, and that would have an effect on the appointment system.

Patients attending for routine check-ups were given ten minutes, and then any treatment required, apart from a quick clean, apportioned a suitable length of time at a later date. That was how things normally worked.

Each morning, a printed 'day list' lay in my surgery, telling me who was coming in when, for what and for how long. A filling appointment might be 20 minutes, an appointment to prepare several teeth for crowns perhaps 90 minutes. Difficult treatments would often be arranged for the end of the session, in case I ran late. Sometimes patients' appointments had to be cancelled at very short notice – or no notice – if a tricky emergency presented itself. If wee Barry fell off his bike and smashed two front teeth it was not a medical emergency, but it most clearly was a dental one, that would require a bit of time to attend to. If patients had to be sent home to accommodate such traumas (a rare event) they always seemed to understand; they were just glad it wasn't them who had gone over the handlebars. Sometimes patients had to be cancelled because the dentist wasn't well. My staff used to relate how patients reacted when they had to be sent away because I had 'Man Flu'.

"I'm sorry Mr Craig has had to cancel all his appointments today as he is unwell."

A look of joyful relief would erupt on their faces. "Oh dear, let's hope it's nothing trivial!"

The busiest times were just before Christmas, or the week before the dentist went off on holiday. I learnt to keep my holiday dates secret. It could be fun meeting a patient coming off the Arran ferry that I was about to board, with my family in tow.

"I'm coming to see you tomorrow with a broken filling."

"No you're not!"

The biggest headache with an appointment system is inadvertent double-booking. Even once fully computerised this could still creep up and try to ruin your day. I had just sat down to spend an hour on Mrs Johnstone's new fillings when I would be told over the intercom that Mr Grinder had appeared for his extraction appointment. I only had one pair of hands: if I had *two* I would have opened in Edinburgh – to almost quote Billy Connolly! The nurse or receptionist would then appear sheepishly at the surgery door to apologise and receive the glare of my 'angry eyes' in return. No matter how we tried to root this problem out, it would rear up to annoy us on a regular basis.

We had an intercom system in the practice and the one in my surgery would come in very handy - apart from its obvious use as a means of informing me of the arrival of patients at the practice or of a telephone call that needed my attention; I always spoke to patients if they phoned in wanting to talk about something – easy access to one's dentist is an important issue, I feel.

We had some fun with the intercom. My nurse could hold the 'talk' button down and we could pretend to have a derogatory conversation about the receptionist. Sometimes the 'talk' button at the receptionist's end would become stuck, and we could hear her chatting about her latest fling to one of the other nurses. It came in very handy at around 1030 each morning, and at frequent intervals thereafter. No tea-breaks were built into our appointment system as we let the staff grab a cuppa whenever they wanted, at an appropriate moment. I used to sip tea almost constantly – my colleague never touched the stuff. Hunger was a daily ordeal to be overcome around 1030 each morning and I had a proclivity for a particular chocolate bar - I am ashamed to admit - the one that was packaged as two separate bars and contained coconut. So I would send out the appeal "is Mr Bond in yet?" A mug of tea would miraculously appear in the staff room. Sometimes my message would be expanded to include: "my next patient is 'bound to' be in, yes?" This led to a tea and the aforementioned chocolate bar appearing in the little staff room a few minutes later.

Communication is critical in practice. I was never sued or ended up in court, yet undeniably over the years I made misjudgements and had treatment failures. Most patients will understand that sometimes things don't always work out as expected. I believe that when something goes wrong then urgent communication and fixing the problem prevents litigation, to put it bluntly. When the new filling you have just carefully crafted falls out, the patient doesn't automatically want to sue you, they just want it fixed – quickly and at no extra cost. That may sound naïve, or maybe I was just lucky, but showing a modicum of sympathy if something isn't right, and then doing the best you can to put it right, is the only way forward. It is up to the dentist, however, to alert the patient to any potential problems that may arise from treating a problem, or indeed *not* treating a problem. A patient may decline a filling, for whatever reason. They should never be coerced into treatment, but warned what might happen if they decline treatment. This would then be written into their records, and when they turn up four months later with a huge abscess the desire to tell them that you told them so ought to be resisted – unless it makes your day to say it!

Confidentiality is fundamental to patient care. Just as in a medical practice, patients are entitled to be frank with their dentist and trust that their personal details, symptoms and treatments aren't blethered at *Sainsburys* or the local pub. I treated many friends, and yes most of them still are, and knew of pregnancies, in-growing toenails and impending divorces well before they became public information. With the development of social media (how I hate that expression) privacy, in all walks of life, has become tested as never before. Maintaining a professional confidentiality when talking to and treating patients within the confines of the surgery was actually easy. There was one simple rule: keep your mouth shut – the dentist that is, the patient had to open theirs.

It was incredible the things some folk would tell you. I was briefed in intimate surgery, bowel movements, affairs, erectile dysfunction and secret admiration of fellow patients in the waiting room. And all that from wee Mr Smith who had just popped in for a denture ease. Which leads me to an important point - one that you may have guessed already. I have shuffled around all the names of patients in this book. When I refer to Mrs Brown, I really mean Ms Green from three doors down. Oh the names are all there – just in a different order, like Eric Morecambe playing the piano.

In return for their lifetime tales, I would retaliate with whatever I wanted to talk about. One advantage of seeing so many people on a daily basis is that you can sway the conversation around to a topic that *you* want to talk about: last night's football, a news item you heard on the radio, my *Rolling Stones* story. Oh have you not heard my *Rolling Stones* story? Well you obviously weren't a patient of mine then!

Despite being very careful with patients' details and records, I can think of one occasion when I let my guard slip. When a patient turns sixteen their parents no longer need to be informed of their child's treatments etc. When a child came into the surgery, leaving mum or dad in the waiting room, I would attend to their needs and then bring the parent into the surgery for an update. If the child turns overnight into a sixteen year old adult, and brings their parent into the surgery, then I assume I can talk to all parties about the treatment, as the young adult has clearly allowed the parent to be present. One morning, Sally, who had just turned sixteen, attended the practice, on her own, with a broken tooth, which I filled. No problem. Later that afternoon her mum came in for a check-up. She casually acknowledged that her daughter had been in that morning to see me.

Clearly not thinking, I blundered "yes, I got her tooth fixed OK."

Now I had been treating Sally since she was knee high to a grasshopper – but she had now turned sixteen, which I had forgotten. Mum said nothing, but went home and asked Sally what was wrong with her tooth, as she thought, incorrectly, that her daughter had perfect teeth. I wasn't privy to the debate that followed but Sally turned up at the practice an hour later and gave me pelters! Why had I told her mum she had a rotten tooth? I hadn't, in so many words, but had as good as. Sally was quite right to be annoyed with me and I humbly apologised, and made sure I checked dates of birth more carefully in future. I had fallen into a trap of my own making.

It was not an uncommon event, actually, for mum and dad to think their little adolescent angel's teeth were immaculate, when I knew otherwise. I learned that day to be more aware of potential errors like that.

A considerable amount of time in a dental practice is spent cleaning and sterilising instruments. Can I just clarify that instruments and items of equipment that are not disposable (and many are) get thoroughly washed and then sterilised in an autoclave. Autoclaves combine heat with pressure to kill all living organisms. They will sterilise and then dry the instruments in just a few minutes, after which they can be packed away in sealable pouches for future use. Within the surgery itself, operating areas and surfaces get wiped with isopropyl alcohol or similar disinfection agents to keep everything squeaky clean; and the dentist has a shower every morning, and at night to get all the bits of dried dentine out of his hair!

All this prevents cross-infection – the inadvertent passage of bacteria and viruses from one patient to another. Dental instruments have always, in modern times, being either properly sterilised or chucked away after use. For many decades dental nurses have also been well schooled in the art and science of cleaning surfaces and chairs etc. But it all takes time and considerable investment to have the sterilising equipment and the duplication of instruments. This was made easier in our practice because we had two autoclaves, and loads of stuff!

The business side of the practice is also time consuming, but in a different way from treating patients. Book work could be done in the evenings, and one of our girls was responsible for handling wages, National Insurances and tax computations.

And then we had to be paid. Each time a patient signs a dental treatment form (normally a GP17) he or she enters a contract with the dentist and the NHS Trust in the area where treatment is being provided. The patient completes the treatment, signs it off and pays 80% of the NHS fee apportioned to all the items of treatment they had carried out. The information on each GP17 is then sent electronically to the Dental Practice Board in Edinburgh, who check it, tally it and eventually authorise the Health Board (trust) to pay the dentist the remaining 20% in a block payment each month, known as a 'schedule'. Patients who are exempt from NHS dental charges have their 80% proportion paid by the Health Board. All NHS treatments have a precise and non-negotiable fee assigned to them – the dentist cannot charge less or more for these items.

The Dental Practice Board basically acts as a go-between and has within its staff dental experts who can advise the dentist on, say, more complicated treatment plans. The Board also conducts random checks on patients who have recently completed a course of NHS treatment. A patient is randomly, apparently, summoned for independent examination by a dentist and a report is sent to the Dental Practice Board and the dentist who carried out the treatment. Sometimes there are comments made which the dentist is required to follow up, and sometimes the dentist just gets a big gold star. It is a fair way of checking that the dentist has carried out the treatment he or she is claiming payment for, and that it has been discharged to a good standard. My only gripe is that the patient is not always made fully aware of *why* this procedure is being undertaken.

Private treatment can be carried out, of course, but the NHS has no influence over this – it is a simple agreement between dentist and patient. The patient agrees a fee and pays it (hopefully).

So dentists in an NHS practice are not actually employed by the health trusts they work under, they take out individual patient contracts though them. In addition to the schedule fees (known as 'item of service fees') dentists also receive payments for the number of patients currently on 'their books'. In return for this various criteria have to be met – which I won't bore you with here. From the total monthly income coming into the practice laboratory fees have to paid to the technicians, materials have to be paid for, staff wages, electricity, insurances, equipment, repairs and so on. Chocolate was the exception – it was paid directly out of the dental nurses' purse. A dental practice is a business – it has to be – and I really enjoyed that aspect of being a dental practitioner.

Sometimes – well quite often actually – patients fail to show up for appointments. As you can imagine this is highly frustrating as time slots are allocated to each procedure. There may be a good reason why someone doesn't show, but often there wasn't. Patients can be rightly charged if they fail an appointment without a reasonable excuse. We sometimes did, but it depended on the circumstances. If wee Mrs Tardy has attended every appointment for the last fifty years then she might be forgiven if she doesn't come through the door for the latest one. She might have died, which is a pretty reasonable excuse, I would say. But when a patient regularly treats their appointment as an inconvenience to the workings of their day, with total disregard for the dentists' time, then he or she will be presented with a bill. That usually stopped the problem or prompted the patient to try out another dentist, which in these circumstances was one of their better ideas.

Some patients loved turning up late, for every appointment; some made a hobby out of it. We would get wise and occasionally retaliate. We had several tools in our armoury for this: we could refuse to see them, we could deliberately give them an appointment time twenty minutes earlier than we expected them, or we could lock the door and put the lights out and pretend we'd gone home. The latter tended not to work "come on Mr Craig, open the door, I know you're in there!"

I heard of an apparently true story, from a few years ago, of a dentist who worked in a practice on the first floor of a tenement property – a common location for dental practices in the west of Scotland. Arriving back from lunch, somewhat late after a harassing morning, he found a queue of patients waiting in the close, outside the locked practice door. Panic rising in his loins he shook his head and announced: "oh he's busy, I'll come back later!"

When I wasn't long qualified, working in Lanarkshire, I became very annoyed one day when a chap whom I had been making a denture for failed to turn up for the fit appointment. He had had a series of appointments and had been a bit late for all of them. When he never showed up at the end of the day I went into a huff, gave him twenty minutes to show and then went home. The next day, one of the practice principals, David, took me aside and explained how the patient had eventually shown up five minutes after I had left. David had seen him and fitted his denture. I was slightly mortified, and then mightily embarrassed. But David explained in his own quiet, proficient manner.

"People are people, Stuart. They will sometimes let you down, but the only way you will get paid for that denture is to swallow your pride and fit it, even if he does arrive late."

It was a lesson I learnt. And of course situations like that can work both ways. The patient can be inconvenienced because their crown hasn't arrived back from the lab at the time you apparently wrote on the lab slip. The dentist is running an hour late, or worse still, is in bed with the 'flu.

Nowadays, with emails and texting, it is much easier to keep tabs on patients and send them little reminders of their appointments. We used to send out 'reminder' letters, informing our patients when their six-month check-ups were due. Many responded like clockwork, coming through the surgery door six months and seven minutes from their previous appointment. Some would phone in, mildly irritated, that they hadn't received their reminder letter on the day they expected it. People like that don't need a letter in the first place. But many folk are remarkably well organised and loyal. When I retired in 2014, I had over a dozen patients whom I had first met back in the Lanarkshire practice thirty-odd years ago. They had followed me from practice to practice - and that is very humbling, I can assure you. Patients *do* like continuity, something which I feel has become rarer in dental practice nowadays. Provided the dentist doesn't treat their mouths like a favourite old car that just needs tinkering with every now and then it is a good relationship: the dentist clearly knows the patient well and recognises their expectations, but the patient also gets to know the dentist; the way they address problems and the relative skills they have. This symbiotic relationship is one that can develop very quickly between dentist and patient and normally works extremely well for both parties. I remember one of those ladies who had been following me from my first practice. She was a very nervous patient, who fortunately needed very little restorative treatment over all those years. But she did break off the side of an upper molar, many visits ago. I wanted to fill it, although it was in a self-cleansing area. She refused, and wanted me to just keep-an-eye on it. At each visit I would offer to fill it, explaining that it would be quite easy and painless to do so. She always refused. I never did get to fill it, but the tooth did not deteriorate and remained symptom free. Had she visited another dentist she might have had her arm twisted a bit further than I had to have it filled, I'm sure, and the new dentist might have wondered why it hadn't been attended to. But such is the nature of some patients' attitudes to treatment. We understood each other well. There is a difference, however, between keeping-an-eye on something and neglect. The interest of the patient always has to come first.

Right, that's some of the boring aspects of running a dental practice explained, let's get to some nitty gritty.

Well all dentists have said that, but sometimes it didn't quite work out that way. Most extractions are a doddle, for both parties involved. Sometimes, however, the dentist finds that a doomed tooth has become belligerent and doesn't want to leave its host as expediently as the dentist anticipated. This can be stressful, as the operator does not want the tooth to win the fight and the tooth's owner wants the procedure to be over as soon as possible, unless they're a masochist.

Extracting teeth can be great fun, I have to admit. There can be a degree of satisfaction in clearing a whole row of loose tombstones, painlessly in under two minutes. Often it took somewhat longer, but then the satisfaction was even greater, especially if the offending ivory flew out and experienced a ricochet off the operating light.

So how are teeth extracted? And this is the bit where you may want to look away, or even leave the room. To remove a tooth we use forceps, not pliers, as patients tend to call them. There are many different types of forceps whose beaks are designed for a particular anatomy of tooth. So there are separate forceps for upper left molars and for upper right molars. Incisors, deciduous teeth, roots, upper wisdom teeth all have their own shape of forceps. The appropriate forceps are chosen and the gum around the tooth is supported by the dentist's gloved fingers. Forceps are gently applied and then eased up, or down, towards the root of the tooth. If the top part of the tooth (crown) only was gripped then the tooth would simply fracture, so the root has to be gripped by the forceps. Teeth are held into their bony sockets by a tough fibrous membrane called the periodontal ligament, but a bit of pushing and wiggling will strip the tooth away from this and it can be gently removed. The socket will naturally bleed, although ingredients in the local anaesthetic reduce this considerably. The socket is gently squeezed to regain its original shape but sutures (stitches) are only needed if there is considerable tearing of the gum, which is sometimes unavoidable. Usually it is as simple as that.

There is an interesting array of other instruments that can be used to extract teeth or roots. Elevators are used to twist roots out. Luxators are a slimmer, sharper version of these that appeared more recently in the dental toolkit. They are used to cut the fibrous periodontal ligament away from the tooth and make it easier to extract. All of these are constructed from shiny steel, as you may recall if you ever watched Bill Murray's obsession with dentist Steve Martin's instruments in the film *Little Shop of Horrors*.

Removing lower permanent molars in adolescents using a type of forcep called *cowhorns* can be a joy. I would argue that cowhorns are one of the best designed dental instruments of all. They have opposing narrow beaks which engage under lower molars. All that is needed is a gentle squeeze and.....pop! For the molar literally pops upwards out of the socket like a champagne cork when the beaks of the cowhorns are gently squeezed together.

Even more fun is when the nicely numbed patient doesn't realise that their tooth is already out. They might think the dentist is just having a final poke around prior to the dastardly deed. I would then step back and ask if they were alright. This would bring a quizzical look to the patient's face. "Is it out?"

"Ages ago, you weren't paying attention."

Some extractions are unintentional. Once, when taking an upper impression of a wee lad, I extracted his loose upper molar. He gave a slight wince when I removed the impression – so did I when I looked at it.

Occasionally the removed tooth has such an enormous root that even the dentist gasps in astonishment.

"Would you like to see *this*?" I might ask the patient, already holding it aloft like a trophy, as if it was the Scottish Cup. And then, to my nurse "don't worry. He'll come round in a minute."

There are times when the dentist can be worried about inadvertently extracting a tooth, or teeth. A patient may present with several loose teeth that require ultimately to be extracted and 'replaced' with a denture, But on taking the impression for the prosthesis there can be a risk of removing a tooth prematurely. The patient would then have a gap during the several days it takes for the technician to fabricate the denture. In these situations the patient has to be well warned.

Fore-warning is being fore-armed – an adage that is very true in dentistry. It can work very well in everyone's favour. Let me give you an example.

An elderly lady needs two lower incisors extracted because they are loose and troublesome. Now elderly ladies, as opposed to elderly men, can bruise very easily with the minimum of trauma. So prior to the extraction it is worth warning the patient that they may develop a bruise on their chin, which might be very noticeable. So if they *do* develop such a bruise, they don't mind because you have told them. A bit of extra foundation will mask it. If they don't develop a bruise they love you because you have clearly been so gentle. But if they get a bruise and you haven't warned them....well you'll be the talk of the steamie.

"Did you see what that dentist did to Aunty Betty? Bruised to her belly button she is."

Some extractions are less fun, however. There can be warning signs. All dentists have become stuck trying to remove a lower wisdom tooth that looked easy on the X-ray. We don't like to give up, you see, but sometimes

31

struggling along with a now fractured wizzie is not the best idea when both patient and dentist are tiring. Lower second premolars can also put up a fight. Teeth do fracture often when being removed. Ideally it is best to get the whole root or roots out, but sometimes this can prove very awkward. The patient can get fed up, or the dentist may have to go for a lie down. Occasionally it is best to just stop, explain to the patient, if they didn't know already, and review the situation at a later date. Usually the patient is content with that. Retained roots tend to become much easier to remove as time goes on. I always tried to resist packing the patient's jaw off to the dental hospital to let someone else have a go.

Being a keen football fan, I used to rearrange some late afternoon appointments around the World Cup schedule, every four years. I remember glancing at the clock just prior to extracting a chap's incisor.

"Will this take long?" He enquired, having spotted me doing this.

"Not at all," I replied, "Holland kick off against Uruguay in fifteen minutes!"

Another chap saw right through me, when the receptionist phoned him to rearrange his 5pm routine check-up.

"....Mr Craig is just running so late this afternoon, we'll have to reappoint." she said apologetically.

"No he isn't, he wants home to see the Scotland Costa Rica game!"

He knew me too well, and I later wished I'd stayed in the surgery.

I am certain that a patient becomes aware when the dentist starts to struggle to remove a troublesome tooth. The practitioner starts to grab all design of steel instruments in an effort to find the one that will finally avulse that last bit of root. Having gone through a whole drawer-full he or she then resorts back to the first one they tried. Patients surely must be aware of this. When the dentist reaches for a spoon or kitchen knife then the patient knows they really are in trouble. A good friend of mine told me that he knew he was in trouble when I started to hum a tune during a hearty extraction. I suppose that had I started belting out Handel's Hallelujah Chorus then he would have asked to leave the room. The same observant friend noted a similar phenomenon when crossing to Islay on CalMac's *Hebridean Isles* a couple of years ago. As the ship started to roll and pitch the crew all donned extra large smiles and started humming as they went about their business; a show of collective reassurance for all passengers to absorb. I suppose it was the same when the band started playing as *Titanic* succumbed.

Anyway, back to teeth. A mentor of mine gave me good advice when getting bogged down in some poor unfortunate's jaw.

"Take a break, give you and the patient a rest. Go swallow a cup of tea, or take an X-ray, if appropriate, then come back and try again."

This invariably worked. Often within seconds the last fragment would be on the floor and there were smiles all around; albeit a lop-sided one from the patient.

Most of the skill in removing awkward teeth is identifying the potentially difficult ones before you even begin. I once numbed a patient prior to extracting an apparently straightforward lower wisdom tooth and then studied the pre-op X-ray one more time. A feeling of impending doom swept over me. I started humming. I decided that caution was the better part of valour – for, you see, dentists don't like to be defeated by a simple wee tooth. I apologised to the patient and explained that I thought that this tooth was going to resist its removal much more that anyone in the room had anticipated: I would refer to the surgical department of Glasgow Dental Hospital. Some weeks later when I saw the patient again I got his end of the ultimate conclusion to this story, and it gave me no pleasure – just a hint of relief – when he related that it had taken the surgeon over an hour to remove it. I didn't always get these decisions right, however.

Things were obviously a lot worse a hundred years ago. It has crossed my mind many times that one of the worst periods in history to be a dental patient was in the years between the discovery of sugar and the invention of local anaesthetics; I leave you to work out the relevant issues yourself.

In the 1937 Journal of the American Dental Association I found a list, complied by a dentist, of "Conditions that cause difficulties in the extraction of teeth." Atop one of the lists, labelled "Unfavourable Patient Attitude" are his examples: bashful and timid, opinionated, careless and lazy, untruthful, foolishly stoical, stupid and (my personal favourite) affected by idiocy. Can you imagine using these expressions today:

"I'm sorry, Mr Smith, I cannot take your tooth out today for I find you a lying, frightened, indolent idiot ....and I've had enough of your stupid opinions."

Sometimes extracted or avulsed (knocked-out) teeth can be transplanted back into the patient's gum. They don't always 'take' but faced with silly Brendan with his front incisor accidently extracted by his mate's beer bottle then it is worth trying. More commonly it is a ten year old who has taken a blow to the face in the school playground. Deciduous teeth would never be reinserted back into their socket but a front permanent incisor that has only been out for a couple of hours, or less, would be a challenge worth undertaking. A good medium for storing the tooth until the patient gets to the dentist is milk; red top, blue top or green top, it doesn't seem to matter. The dentist can try to insert it back into the socket gently and splint (glue) it to adjacent teeth for a few days. Very often a successful result will ensue, although the tooth will probably have to be root-treated at a later date.

I found an early example of a similar kind of re-implantation in the British Dental Journal (BDJ) of 1894. A robust 17 year old had presented with an upper premolar with a large decayed cavity in it. The tooth was removed and cleaned with a weak solution of phenolic acid. The following morning the pulp (nerve) was removed and it was root-treated and filled with amalgam. It was then placed back in the socket, where four months later it still remained, apparently functional.

Transplanting other people's teeth into a different individual still remains fanciful, I'm afraid. Maybe one day it will be possible: "can I have Ken Dodds' teeth please?" Although the idea of transplantation between different people is not a new one. There was once a profitable trade where rich and edentulous (having no natural teeth) 'patients' could opt for having the freshly extracted teeth of criminals stuck into their jaws. I wonder whose ordeal was the worst – the donor or the recipient, especially when the reimplanted tooth fell out a few days later.

In more recent times it was very common to have all of one's teeth removed as a forthcoming birthday present or family event – usually a 21st or a wedding. These were the days before NHS funding of dental treatment, and those with poor teeth could ill afford dental bills. The easier answer was a 'clearance' – the removal of the whole lot, followed by the fitting of immediate full dentures. It seems socially reprehensible now, but was common place not so long ago, and perfectly acceptable to the patient. Imagine the delight to the groom if on receiving his new dentures he finds his bride has gone through the same procedure and arrives at the top of the aisle with a gleaming new set too. Throughout their future partnership their respective dentures could sit and smile at each other through their glass tumblers at their bedside. That's true love.

Clearances are still performed, unfortunately, in cases where there is such neglect that there is no restorative option. I think the most teeth I ever removed in one sitting, under local anaesthetic, was sixteen. But with the development of bridges and implants the provision of 'immediate' dentures is less common. Even the word 'clearance' sounds extreme. Wholesale extraction of teeth to replace them with fresh, white replacements is redolent of the Highland Clearances, where people were forcibly evicted and substituted with white things – sheep.

Extraction sockets are usually remarkably free of pain, especially when you consider what a similar wound on, say, your arm would feel like - indeed sockets in young children often require no analgesics as they just don't seem to hurt. The exception is when the socket becomes a 'dry socket'. This is when, for obscure reasons, the blood clot in the socket disintegrates and the bony walls of the socket are exposed. This can cause an exceedingly painful gum, which antibiotics will not help and which will linger for up to ten days. The dentist can pack the socket frequently to relieve the discomfort but it is an unpleasant phenomenon.

To avoid problems with sockets the patient is advised to rinse frequently with hot, salty water, 24 hours after the extraction. Allowing this time for the blood clot in the socket to settle, hot, salty mouthwashes really do keep the socket and clot clean and less likely to become infected. The heat improves the blood supply to the area, promoting speedy healing, and the salt has considerable anti-bacterial properties. When reviewing a patient a few days after an extraction I could always tell if the patient had been doing as they were told and using the mouthwash.

Clearly some teeth are easier to extract than others. Upper canines can be tricky as they have very long elliptical roots. Most big lower molars are easy - especially if amenable to cowhorns – and some upper molars are trickier, as they have three roots. Inevitably the dentist may really struggle to remove a tooth –we've all been there many times. I can remember trying to extract an upper molar from a big-jawed chap many years ago. I just could not budge it. It didn't break, but it didn't move either. After several minutes we both agreed to stop, but I hit on a plan. I sent him away with painkillers and reappointed him the next day. I reckoned all that pushing and twisting would 'soften up' the periodontal ligament. Surprisingly, the chap showed up the next day, and the tooth came out at the first tug.

Apart from extractions undertaken in patients' homes, as explained further on, I've also removed teeth from my own children at home. Not because they were naughty, it's normally their toe-nails we removed for that, but for planned orthodontic reasons. There was one notable exception. I extracted my daughter Fiona's baby incisor aboard paddle steamer *Waverley*. It was very loose and it was bothering her. So a small wedge of ice from the bar ice-bucket helped freeze the gum and clean fore finger and thumb did the rest. She wasn't interested in putting it under her pillow however, so it now rests in the depths of the Clyde, somewhere between Dunoon and Rothesay.

Dentists are generally never keen to extract a tooth if it can be otherwise restored. To be frank, they get a bigger fee for restorative work than demolition work, so why get rid of it? There are times though when the best advice is extraction. Ultimately the dentist can only advise, but the patient has the power of veto, as with any treatment of course. After all, it is their tooth! Many times I would suggest an extraction and the patient would decline. That is all very well, as long as the dentist has explained why it should be removed and any potential outcomes of leaving it – such as infection, further fracture etc. One lady thought carefully about my recommendation and suggested we just leave well alone. "I think I'll just keep it, it seems a bit like putting a dog down while it's still wagging its tail." I couldn't disagree with her.

I had one young woman, many years ago, that agreed to the extraction but didn't want a numbing injection. I tried to persuade her that it would be intolerably painful, but she insisted I go ahead. I knew she would change her mind, so applied the forceps very gently; and then squeezed the handles. She changed her mind very quickly after that!

I have never knowingly extracted the wrong tooth. I may have removed one only to discover, when the patient returned a few days later, that there was another problem, or that the patient's symptoms had been somewhat misrepresented. That is forgivable – we are not super human. I did hear of a situation, however, where the dentist did make an error. The patient was a labourer who attended the practice in pain. The dentist diagnosed correctly and numbed upper left first premolar, with a view to its extraction. As she was having a busy morning she sent the chap out to the waiting room to give the anaesthetic some time to work. Fifteen minutes later she called him back in and extracted his tooth. He never flinched, but asked curiously at the end, why she had numbed the left hand side but extracted a tooth from the right hand side! Perhaps she had forgotten to do the wee pin test with a sharp probe before commencing.

Some folk have been known to extract their own teeth in desperation – non-dentist folk, I mean, although I have heard of one dentist who extracted his own tooth. You would be forgiven for thinking that the sensible thing to do would be to just to go to a dentist, for they generally know how to do it. But sometimes fear or opportunity takes over. Maybe the tooth was so loose it could be pushed back and forth with the tongue. Even so, to tease it away from that last wee bit of tenacious gum is not easy – and not painless. A terminally loose tooth will eventually fall out, but it can take a long time.

When I worked in Lanarkshire the practice was occasionally visited by seamen from ships that had docked at Glasgow. Many were Filipinos, Singaporeans or Chinese, and they were in need of urgent dental treatment. Here I saw an entire atlas of dentistry - eastern style. Lots of gold crowns and shoogly bridges. Some of these chaps needed an extraction, some had already had one, courtesy of one of their ship mates. Usually they could speak no English, and my Mandarin is unreliable, but with the help of a translator, or sign language, we got them sorted. It was touching to have your hand gripped and receive a now toothless smile in gratitude; after all these poor chaps may have been suffering for weeks.

Deciduous (baby) teeth fall out naturally because the roots dissolve (resorb) away as the permanent tooth underneath pushes through from under it. Parents often brought wee Maggie's incisor in for me to check where the root was. Was it still in the gum? No it has resorbed, thus allowing the tooth to loosen and fall out. Another source of puzzlement was what happens to back deciduous teeth. Do they fall out? Of course they do, by the same process, but by then the child is older, the tooth less noticeable as it is at the back of the mouth, and less fuss is made. I have a brother-in-law who, on completion of his own curry with boiled rice, proceeded to finish off his six year old son's leftovers. Crunch! He bit down on something hard. It wasn't a grain of basmati, it was the wee chap's lower incisor, which he had just plucked out and left at the side of his plate.

"Dentist! Av goat the pyorrhoea. Ma gums are killing me!"

Literally 'pyorrhoea' means 'flow of pus' (how nice) but what is this mysterious disease? In truth it does exist, less commonly now, but is a term which has gone out of fashion for advanced gum disease and what the dental profession call 'acute ulcerative gingivitis'. The latter is not the run-of-the-mill gum inflammation that everyone gets sometimes – and some people have all the time – this is a specific infection caused by a couple of not very friendly bacteria. Left untreated it will cause permanent loss of the architecture of the gum around the teeth (gingivae) and in theory, if totally neglected, could mean your gums do indeed kill you.

It is not so common nowadays but is generally caused by poor oral hygiene and smoking. You cannot catch it from a dirty beer glass or coffee mug and dentists can spot and treat it, with antibiotics, very quickly. Unlike general gingivitis (gum inflammation) this type of gum infection is painful, and smelly. Dentists can often diagnose it before they look in the mouth, just by walking into the waiting room, closing their eyes and sniffing. "Oh I can tell Mr Brown's in again, oh and we have a case of ulcerative gingivitis too."

The commoner gum disease I was referring to is the progressive loss of the supporting tissues of the teeth due to gingivitis and ultimately periodontitis (inflammation of the deeper supporting tissues). This I discuss in a later chapter. Antibiotics will not help this type of periodontitis.

The mouth is remarkably resistant to infection. Further back the throat succumbs to all sorts of viral and bacterial infection, but not the mouth. With the exception of fungal and viral infections any infection in the mouth is almost always associated with a tooth, or teeth.

There is a whole kaleidoscope of other colourful oral diseases and afflictions to which people can succumb, but thankfully these are not common. Some arthritic type of conditions can affect the mouth, as can a few bone conditions, but these are rare.

Scurvy is now unheard of but back in the days of Jolly Jack Tar, before it was realised that it was a lack of vitamin C from fresh fruit and vegetables that was causing it, scurvy killed scores of sailors. Vitamin C is essential for, among other things, maintaining connective tissue – the fibrous stuff that joins all our bits together, and glues our teeth in. One of the first manifestations of scurvy, then, was when the poor chap's teeth fell out and were left embedded in the hard tack or salted beef that he was biting into. Had he been biting into an apple the same thing would have happened – but then if he was biting into an apple he wouldn't have had scurvy. Thanks in part to a Scottish doctor James Lind, who conducted one of the world's first clinical trial while at sea on the Bay of Biscay, scurvy became effectively confined to history in just a few years. In my career I never saw scurvy, not that I was likely to, although I sailed on paddle steamer *Waverley* many times. In fact the vast majority of oral diseases in the encyclopaedia I never saw, thankfully. As an undergraduate the oral medicine professor did try to catch me out, however. As I walked past his surgery one afternoon he grabbed me inside and pointed to the young lad in his chair.

"Mr Craig, have a look at this lad's tongue and give me a provisional diagnosis."

I took a mouth mirror, and gently peered into the chap's mouth. Everything looked normal, except for his tongue; it was bright purple.

"What do you think is going on here, Mr Craig?" Asked the Prof.

Spotting the wrapper hanging out of the lad's pocket I replied assuredly.

"I think he's been eating a purple lollipop, Professor."

The Prof laughed, so did the patient, and I banked the Brownie Points – just in case I needed them at a future, more conventional, student examination.

A very common oral condition that most of us have suffered from at one time or another is *aphthae* or common ulcers. These circular, greyish little beasts occur on the inside of the lips, at the back of a row of teeth and on the side of the tongue and can be very painful. They are commoner in young adults, when they sometimes appear in two's and three's. They are harmless but a real *pain* literally. Their cause is not clear, although they can be linked to hormonal changes, such as menstruation, and to stress. Over time they tend to stop appearing, but patients shouldn't hesitate to speak to their dentist if they suffer regularly from them or if they appear as larger ulcers. There are medications that the dentist can prescribe to help.

Ulcers also occur due to viral infections - usually in very painful clusters - in children or young adults, but in these cases the patients generally feel unwell. The causative agent here is usually a herpes infection, and they can be contagious. I remember treating three chaps with this condition over the course of a week. I puzzled as to the link, and then discovered they all drank in the same pub. Maybe it was just a coincidence, but nevertheless this type of cross infection is very rare.

Naturally the one oral condition that does concern some patients is oral cancer, which can also present as an ulcer. In these cases, however, the ulcer does not heal over a week or two but persists. Oral cancer usually affects the soft tissues such as under the tongue or behind the last molars. It is not common, but becoming commoner, for reasons which are not entirely clear. Dentists are in the perfect position to screen for oral cancer and are well trained in spotting it. Anyone concerned about an unusual swelling, ulcer or white patch anywhere in their mouth should see their dentist as soon as they can. Usually it will not be a cancer. In my 38 years I saw just three oral cancers. All were in soft tissue. One was being treated regularly and successfully, one I picked up very early on and likewise was kept well under control. The third was devastatingly advanced, in a 46 year old man who had sadly ignored the warning signs for eighteen months and never visited a dentist. This was in my first year of qualification and I was quite shocked to find something which looked just like the lesions that had stared out of the textbook at me. I had the patient seen at Glasgow Dental Hospital the next day. He had surgery but sadly died some four months later.

So please, don't worry about oral cancer, but get regular check-ups from your family dentist - even if you wear full dentures. Your dentist will always routinely examine all of your mouth at check-up. Many patients are well tuned-in to this and I regular saw edentulous (having no natural teeth) patients for a check-up. It takes just a couple of minutes and I could see the relief on the faces of many people when I reassured them that their mouth was perfectly fine - apart from not having any teeth! Many ladies with full dentures were clearly embarrassed to be seen without their dentures - even by their dentist. I can clearly understand that. I would reassure them that I couldn't give a jot; I was just doing my health care professional bit - just like their gynaecologist! Actually, I didn't add that last bit, for we can all suffer from embarrassment when confronted with intimate examinations. It was quite common to learn that their husband never saw them without their dentures - so I was privileged.

Talking of gynaecologists (were we?) I heard a good tale, probably apocryphal, of the female dentist who visited her 'gynae' for a minor procedure. Making idle chat, the doctor asked his patient what she worked at.

"I'm a dentist."

"Goodness, do you not get fed up looking into patients' mouths all day?"

It wasn't uncommon for a patient to look in the mirror one morning, peer at their mouth, spot something they didn't like and come rushing down to the surgery in a minor panic. My receptionist always told them to have a seat and I would see them within a few minutes to reassure them that what they were looking at was either a normal feature, a piece of wedged tomato skin or a stuck haddock bone. I can remember one lady in a terrible state of nerves - she had spotted a bluish swelling at the side of her tongue, quite far back. I will never forget the look of relief when I pointed out that these were just large veins, that they were perfectly normal and that she had a similar set on the other side of her tongue. She hadn't looked at the other side of her mouth. In all these anxious people - who quite rightly wanted to get checked, by the way - I never found a single suspicious lesion.

A common cause of alarm is when the patient notices, surprisingly for the first time, the row of very large red, raised papillae – like swollen taste buds – that lie just over the horizon on the surface of the tongue. These are called 'circumvallate papillae' and are perfectly normal. Because they are almost out of sight it is perhaps not surprising that people don't notice them unless they take a mouth mirror to the back of their mouth.

There are quite a number of systemic conditions, affecting other parts of the body but unrelated to teeth, which can manifest in the mouth. This is one of the reasons dentists are well trained in general pathology, medicine and pharmacology. Among the diseases which can be suspected by a dentist are: diabetes, kidney disease, neurological problems, leukaemia, AIDS, bone disorders, anaemia, auto-immune diseases and even pregnancy and depression. Over my career I saw patients with oral manifestations of all of these conditions (with the exception of leukaemia).

When I was a student AIDS was just beginning to be identified as the devastating disease it is. You will all be relieved to hear that the excellent hygiene measures that were already in place prevented any risk of the HIV virus being spread in dental practice. Catching an infection from another patient, or dental staff, in a dental surgery just doesn't happen. So when AIDS became the new plague that was going to threaten us all, dentists really had to make no or little alteration to their normal hygiene practice. Only one patient ever asked me if I used a different injection needle for each patient. He seemed pleasantly surprised when I said 'of course'. Not only is the needle disposed of, but so is the glass cartridge holding the local anaesthetic, and root-treatment instruments, polishing brushes, mouth-wash cups, suction tubes...I could go on and on.

The issue with cross infection is not the patient with AIDS or hepatitis, it is the patient who nobody knows has such an infectious disease. Therefore all patients are treated as an infection risk. I only knowingly saw one patient with AIDS. He was a lad of about twenty who attended the practice in order to get a new partial denture made. He looked ill but not particularly frail. I took the necessary impressions and gave him three further appointments, a week apart. The following week he never showed up, so our receptionist gave his home a call to find out why. He had died a couple of days after visiting the practice.

I mentioned that we had received a lot of training in general medicine. Apart from lectures at the university this had involved ward visits, to medical and surgical wards, at Glasgow's Royal Infirmary. I loved these. We learned so much about the human condition and the diseases that are often inflicted upon us. The doctors and surgeons gave us the same respect as they gave to the medical students and we tended to hold them in a bit of awe. The vast majority of problems we saw were not dental; as my surgical ward was in the liver and gastro-intestinal department I became an expert on duodenal ulcers, obstructive jaundice and alcoholic liver disease!

Apart from learning about medicine, these ward visits were designed to teach us how to examine a patient and how to ask the right questions. The patients usually thought we were medical students, and when they were told we were dentals, as they sometimes were, they would frequently ask "Why do you need to know all that stuff just to pull teeth out?" However, lying in a hospital bed, bored and perhaps feeling unloved most patients seemed to thoroughly enjoy the little group of students that popped around to see them of a Wednesday morning. Especially as their surgeon was in attendance too. After all, they got to tell us all about their symptoms and watch our faces as we tried to guess what ailed them. I think in some cases the surgeon or ward sister had been just ahead of us, asking the patients not to give too much away. This led to some interesting answers as we honed down our questioning and diagnosis skills.

"Tell me Mr Anderson," one of my colleagues asked, "what brought you here?"

"It was a number 38 bus, son?"

I can recall one amusing case where it was me that was doing the examination. The lady was in her late forties and she had an enlarged liver. Our surgeon, Mr Joffe, indicated that I should examine the patient and enquire into her symptoms. By this time we had spent a few weeks in wards so I considered that I knew how to palpate an enlarged liver.

"Do you mind if I feel your liver?" I asked gingerly.

The lady pulled her gown up to her shoulders, "carry on."

I felt under the right hand side of her rib cage, just as I had been shown.

"Mmm, I see," I mumbled, in my best Dr Cameron voice.

The lady looked up at me. "So, when will you be a doctor?"

I looked back at her. "I'm not going to be a doctor, I'm going to be a dentist."

She immediately pulled her gown back down – and that was the end of the examination. I wonder what she said to the surgeon afterwards.

We saw things that we would never see again in our collective careers. Burns, stomas, tumours, and we met a lot of lovely people. Some of the many patients I saw left an indelible impression on me. I can recall our small group of six being ushered into a small private room to talk to a fifty year old chap who was sitting on a chair beside his bed. The right hand side of his face looked floppy, as if he had suffered a stroke. We were encouraged to ask questions. He told us that over the course of a couple of weeks the right side of his face had become weak – clearly a dentally orientated condition. He seemed cheerful enough and happy to talk to us.

The physician then thanked him and ushered us into a nearby room where two radiographs were being illuminated: one a chest X-ray and the other a head X-ray. The poor chap had lung cancer, with secondary deposits in the part of the brain that dealt with facial muscle control. He was incurably ill, but didn't yet know. I felt terrible for him.

One by-product of all these ward rounds was that every student, me included, started to imagine there was a fair degree of pathology going on in our own bodies. I was certain I had a tummy ulcer and one of the guys was sure he had syphilis - actually, it wouldn't have been a surprise if he had, come to think! A twitch in an eyebrow was interpreted as the onset of a stroke. Not going to the toilet for two consecutive days was heralding bowel cancer. That pimple under the arm can only mean Hodgkin's Disease! Was that a touch of yellow in the whites of the eyes?

I do believe that the year we spent visiting the Royal, three mornings a week, turned the tide into converting us from adolescent students into professional people, with an empathy for patients who suffered from problems that we didn't have.

GETTING STRAIGHTENED OUT

My stock advice to teenage patients with squinty teeth was: "I'll refer you to an orthodontist colleague of mine – he'll straighten you out." A fair number of teenagers need straightened out, you won't be surprised to hear. I really mean their teeth need straightened, of course. Orthodontics is the art and science of achieving that; of straightening teeth. *Ortho* is from the Greek word meaning 'straight or upright'. Baby (deciduous) teeth don't need straightened, even if they seem a bit short of space in the jaws. Crooked deciduous teeth, however, are a reasonable indication that the second, permanent teeth may be short of space when they erupt into the mouth. So orthodontics really applies to the permanent dentition.

The process of tooth eruption is one of life's mysteries, like bird migration, Harry S. Truman's middle name or what Captain Mainwaring's wife looks like. Teeth tend to want to get into the correct position, on their own accord, but just how is still a bit of a puzzle. Perhaps they navigate with the help of the stars, like the birds. The 'stars' certainly have an influence on the demand for orthodontic treatment – many young people want their smiles to look like the gleaming ramrod straight piano keys of their Hollywood and TV idols. On the waiting room wall of the last practice I worked in was a television which occasionally threw up some famous faces *before* and *after* their dental refurbishment – although clearly not at our practice. One of these was Tom Cruise. One day one of my patients came in and pointed enthusiastically at the telly.

"I'd be happy with the '*before*' appearance if you could manage that."

So why bother straightening teeth? One may justifiably ask. Well lots of good reasons, actually. If teeth are misaligned they don't look so pleasing, are more difficult to clean and can cause problems such as gum disease, difficult occlusion (bite) and future restorative issues. In days gone by a removable appliance was fitted to tilt the teeth into a better position, usually after sacrificing a couple of adjacent teeth in order to create the necessary space. This works in limited situations but nowadays fixed appliances are used, where brackets are cemented to the teeth and wires passed along the brackets to physically pull the teeth into the desired position. Fixed appliances work better for they can exert a greater degree of torque to the teeth and can thus pull them along instead of merely tilting them. They have another overriding advantage – the patient can't take them out so they work 24/7.

The commonest reason for needing orthodontic treatment is crowding (not overcrowding). That is, insufficient space for the last permanent teeth to appear to erupt into. This usually involves the canine teeth in the upper jaw (arch) and second premolar teeth in the lower – simply because these tardy individuals are the last to arrive. Parents used to state that their little darlings had too many teeth. This is exceptionally rare, so I would correct them: "he has precisely the right number of teeth, but not enough space for them all right now." The reasons for crowding we won't go into here, but it could have something to do with the notion that we were designed to eat a coarser diet and thus wear our teeth down at the points where they contact each other, thus creating more space for subsequent tooth eruption.

There are lots of other reasons why orthodontic treatment is recommended, such as a disparity between the jaws and functional reasons, but we won't go into that either.

I wore a URA (upper removable appliance) when I was about 16. I always took it out when meeting my girlfriend – she never knew I wore one, and never noticed my canines gradually swinging nicely into line. There was a real panic one day when I unexpectedly met her on a number 59 bus in Kelvindale. Much coughing, turning my head away and playing about with a scarf ensured that she remained in orthodontic ignorance.

Sometimes teeth become gradually pushed forwards, or indeed backwards, by the action of the soft tissues such as lips and tongues. A lower lip being frequently jammed under protruding upper teeth will serve to compound he situation, and perhaps result in the patient looking a touch like *Plug*, that famous *Bash Street Kid* - from The Beano. Those clever orthodontists can fix this, of course, but sometimes a child may have a habit which only adds to the problem. Thumb-sucking, or more accurately digit-sucking, can push protruding teeth out further. Kids can invent all sorts of ingenious ways to stick their fingers into their mouths and make the orthodontist's work that bit more difficult. It could be a thumb, a forefinger or a whole row of fingers turned around 180 degrees and stuffed in. It may give comfort to the child but can cause grief for the dentist. When a child uses their fingers as a comfort before they develop their permanent incisors (say about 7) this is rarely a problem. When they stop the habit the teeth and supporting bone recover to their normal position. But when the child is older they should really be encouraged to stop. This can be with gentle persuasion, the wearing of an appliance with a hole cut in the palate of the plate to prevent suction, a programme of orthodontic treatment or even more drastic measures – such as cutting their fingers off.

Children, being the inventive creatures that they are, can insert lots of other non-anatomical objects into their faces to try to prise their teeth forwards: pens, pencils, someone else's digits. So, on examining wee ones where I suspected such a habit it was worth asking them if they liked to partake in such activities. I remember one smart wee lassie who seemed receptive to such gentle cross examination.

"What nice teeth you have, Kylie. Tell me, do you suck your thumb?"

"No."

"Chew your pencil at school?"

"Nope."

But I've clearly got her thinking. ".....but I twiddle my hair!"

On a separate occasion the conversation was remarkably similar.

"Tell me Brendan, do you suck your fingers or chew your pencil at school?"

"No."

"Do you bite your nails?"

"No." But this wee lad was really getting tuned to the same wavelength. "No, but I pick my toes."

I am a big fan of orthodontic treatment. It works! If offered by your dentist I suggest you consider it, after being informed of the options, of course. There are few risks if treated properly, and in my experience it was always performed properly by highly skilled orthodontists. One most important part of orthodontic treatment cannot, however, be understated. RETENTION. Once active treatment is over another type of appliance (a retainer) has to be worn to allow the teeth to settle down. Usually this is worn for 6-12 months. This is because the teeth that have been moved, having been repositioned against their will, have a strong desire, like young salmon, to return to their starting positions. If wee Mary doesn't wear her retainers then years of work can speedily become undone. So, wear the retainers!

Sometimes Plug himself would walk into the surgery and proclaim that he wanted to look like Janet Street Porter or perhaps slightly better. Yes, orthodontic treatment also works for adults but generally takes longer, has to be retained for a longer period afterwards and costs more, as it will not be funded by the NHS. Generally, unless they really *do* look like *Plug*, I would encourage patients asking about ortho treatment to visit the expert and, if treatment is recommended, to go for it. Usually the results were terrific, although some patience was required and a few grand in the bank desirable.

One of the concerns of parents, and perhaps even more so by the patient, is that teeth usually have to be sacrificed at the start of orthodontic treatment.

"What! Second teeth are being extracted! Four of them!"

This is not a problem in itself. Space has to be created once the permanent teeth have appeared. The teeth further forward are then aligned into this space. These extractions have to be balanced, the same number on either side of the mouth, otherwise the final result will all sit to the one side - like Gourock. Often teeth will also have to be removed in the opposing arch of teeth. This is why it is often four teeth which are sacrificed. Usually premolar teeth are the victims as there are loads of them and they don't look particularly pretty anyhow.

The privilege of extracting the teeth always falls to the child's usual dentist – I must have removed hundreds of them. Often the child has good teeth, and therefore this is the first surgical intervention they have ever had in their mouths, and perhaps anywhere else. So one can imagine the scene, when little Freddy appears at the surgery, pale and worried-looking at 9 in the morning to have four teeth out. Sometimes it took all of my persuasive powers but over the years I've got to hand it to these youngsters, they usually took it in their stride. In fact these extractions are very easy for both dentist and patient as the chosen teeth submit themselves painlessly and speedily to the forceps. Having said that, I hated doing ortho extractions and would always split it into two sessions, much to the annoyance sometimes of the attending parent who wanted the whole experience over in one go. Funnily enough, the young patient was usually more than happy to split the procedure, and so got their wish. Inevitably their nerves had subsided on the second visit as they now knew just how easy it all was the first time around. Usually I would donate the extracted teeth to the patient as they left (although the health authorities don't seem to like this idea nowadays) after a obtaining a promise from the patient that they wouldn't try to reinsert them.

Which reminds me of an early incident when I worked in Lanarkshire not long after qualifying. I had to perform two extractions from a well-behaved lad of about ten years of age - let's call him Freddy. I removed a decayed lower permanent molar first of all. The trickiest one over, I then proceeded to work on the loose but troublesome deciduous molar directly above the now oozing socket. Out it popped like a pearly champagne cork (they often do) and immediately vanished from sight. After a look around the mouth, the patient's clothes, the dental nurse's uniform and the floor of the surgery the tooth could not be found. Having satisfied myself that the lad hadn't swallowed (or worse, inhaled) the small tooth I explained the situation to his mum and sent them on their way. A further search of my chair and goldfish tank failed to illicit what had happened to the baby tooth and no more was thought about it.

Eight months elapsed and Freddy appeared at the surgery for his routine check-up. Lo and behold what is this? Appearing out of the now healed socket where his permanent lower molar had once been, is a new tooth. It looks exactly like an upper first deciduous molar, only it is back to front! When I extracted the baby molar it had fallen into the socket I had created on taking the lower permanent molar out. Over the ensuing months this had now tried to erupt into the mouth, pretending to be a new tooth and now presented itself, the wrong way round! The other dentists in the practice thought this was hilarious, but not so Freddy who had to have his tooth removed for the second time!

As any Glaswegian will tell you "wally" means china or porcelain. *Wally* comes from 'wall' as the walls of the entrance hallways (closes) of Glasgow tenements were tiled with porcelain tiles. The 'posher' the close the fancier the tile used.

As dentures, or false-teeth, were originally made out of porcelain (they tend to be made of acrylic now) then it was completely understandable that they would soon be known as 'wallies' – being the natural plural of wally. It is an expression still in parlance today. So as Stanley Baxter would say: "I cannae find ma wallies" would be accurately translated as "Has anyone seen my full upper and lower dentures?"

Dentists never refer to 'false-teeth'. The correct term is denture, whether it is a full denture or a partial denture, and the science of denture prescription and construction is known as prosthodontics; sometimes shortened to prosthetics.

At one time, in the not too distant past, over 40% of adults in Glasgow over 16 years of age possessed not a single natural tooth. A shameful statistic but the root cause of which (please excuse the pun) I will not go into here for I am not writing a social history. As a result of this dentists qualifying from Glasgow, in particular, around the time I qualified and the years immediately before me, were pretty good at making dentures – because they had lots of practice. When I started work in Lanarkshire in 1981 I would usually have about a dozen full denture patients on-the-go at any one time. Things have improved, thankfully. My dentist daughter probably makes one set every three months.

Dentures, as I said, are now constructed out of acrylic – both the plate part and the actual artificial teeth. For the plate (base) of the denture the acrylic comes in the form of a powder/liquid mix which is cured in an oven. Before acrylic they were made out of wood, or ivory and then vulcanite.

Vulcanite is a type of flexible rubber, invented by Mr Charles Goodyear, of tyre fame, in 1843. Once porcelain teeth could be fixed into the vulcanite, a handful of years later, dentures could be made more cheaply. Its main drawback was the dark colour of the vulcanite and the propensity for the porcelain teeth to fall out. There are also rare supposed cases of vulcanite causing symptoms of toxicity. Dentist Mr Newton Petit describes in the British Dental Journal of 1892 a female patient of his suffering 'mercurial' poisoning as soon as the dentures were inserted in her mouth, which ceased as soon as they were removed. This gives some authority to the patient struggling into the surgery with their newly fitted dentures proclaiming "Ma wallies are killing me!"

Despite this, vulcanite was in widespread use for denture bases until superseded by acrylic in the late 1930s. I well remember elderly patients coming in with vulcanite dentures, which by the 1980s were looking a bit the worse for wear. I recall one very old lady bringing her vulcanite denture in for repair.

"How old is this?" I asked tentatively, holding the denture between thumb and forefinger at arm's length.

"I got it just before the war," she mumbled.

"Goodness, so it's about fifty years old then?"

"Oh no son," she retorted, "the *first* war!"

The story of the use of vulcanite in dentistry is an interesting one with a rather nefarious twist to it: enter stage right – one Samuel Chalfont.....and then he can leave again, for he crops up in a later chapter.

A lot of denture provision is for replacement dentures. I would advise a new set every six or seven years; some patients would want a new set more frequently. I loved denture work; it could be very rewarding, giving the patient a new smile or restoring their old one. There is quite a craft to denture construction though, and the relationship between dentist and the technician - who is ultimately going to make them - is fundamental and crucial.

Taking the construction of full dentures as an example - the dentist firstly takes the impressions of upper and lower gums. Sometimes a second set of impressions is taken for greater accuracy, using impression trays that have been constructed from the casts of the patient's mouth from the first impression. The technician then makes wax 'bite blocks' that fit the plaster casts of the mouth. These are tried in the mouth at the next visit, known as the jaw registration, and various parameters are cut into the wax, such as the occlusion (bite) between the blocks, the tooth position, the height and size of the teeth, and so on. When one of our nurses sat her dental nursing exam a few years ago she gave an audacious reply to one of the questions on dentures. When asked what materials she needed to look out for a 'jaw registration appointment' she replied: "kettle, cup, tea bag, milk."

And when asked to explain her answer she said: "well, we usually go for a cup of tea when the dentist is doing the jaw registration." She did actually pass the exam.

Anyway, back to denture design. From the altered wax blocks the technician now sets up the teeth in the wax and these are tried-in at the next clinical visit. The patient gets a chance to see them at this visit – unless they run down two inches from one side to the other, or the teeth chosen by the dentist make the patient look like *Shergar*. Alterations can then be made and the trial dentures either 're-tried' at the next appointment or completed by the technician and fitted at the final visit. Wax is the ideal medium for holding the teeth in place temporarily. When I was a student, one of my colleagues had a lady in the prosthetics clinic for a 'try-in' of her wax dentures. She asked if she could pop out to the waiting room to show her husband her new look. Unfortunately, having showed him they then decided to nip down to the cafeteria for a cup of tea. She spent the next half hour spitting out teeth.

Once the dentist and patient are happy with the try-in dentures they head back to the technician. He or she then embeds the dentures in plaster, in a metal flask. Once the plaster is set, the flask is opened and the wax is removed using boiling water. This leaves a void in the plaster corresponding to the shape of the 'gum' part of the denture, with the teeth embedded in the plaster. Acrylic is mixed and placed where the wax was, and the flask is then cooked in an oven to cure the acrylic. The flask is opened, the plaster smashed way and the acrylic denture is trimmed and polished.

The construction of a partial denture is similar. It must be realised that the technician constructs the dentures to the design (prescription) given by the dentist. And believe me, dental technicians are highly skilled people. When I started my own practice I was advised at a seminar that the first bill the dentist should pay each month was his technician's. I can honestly say I always did.

Patients seem to dread getting impressions taken. Certainly, in the days when good old drippy plaster of Paris was used it often caused much retching in the sensitive palate. But modern impression materials are excellent and even in sensitive mouths most patients find getting an impression taken, whether it's for a denture or a crown or to make a simple model of their mouth, is really quite easy.

Being not too keen on the sight of 'puke' I tried early on to perfect the technique of impression taking. It is a bit like driving a car. It seems very tricky to begin with and the result is often squinty, but with practice it becomes easy to achieve a good impression. Trying not to make the patient sick was high up in my list of criteria and in my years of practice I only failed to prevent that twice – and one of them was an eight year old (no I wasn't making dentures for them!)

As I said, many of the dentures being made were replacements and I can think back to some lovely patients for whom I made four or five sets during my career. Some couldn't care less what the final outcome looked like. Others were more particular. Most of the time everything worked out fine. Sometimes it didn't and I was forced into expensive re-makes or alterations to put things right.

Particular anatomical features can make life tricky for both dentist and technician. I found an article in the 1937 Journal of The American Dental Association referring to a poor chap suffering from acromegaly as being

"...a prosthetic monstrosity." Acromegaly is a rare hormonal disease which leads to certain bones expanding in adulthood; the lower jaw (mandible) is often involved. When working in Lanarkshire I had a gentleman whose lower jaw protruded about 5 cm in front of his upper. He was not suffering from acromegaly, he just had a big jaw, a bit like *Shrek*, come to think. Normally the relationship between the jaws is such that the upper jaw protrudes a bit more than the lower, but a 'reverse bite' (or class lll, as it is referred to) is pretty common. However in Mr Smith's case it was extreme, and no matter how much I wanted to place his lower denture teeth inside his uppers, or indeed inside his mouth, there was no way that it was going to be easy. His lower jaw stuck out so much that he was in constant danger of drowning whenever it rained. I sought the advice of the technician, who lived locally.

"Oh no, you've got Jimmy Smith, I dreaded the day I would have to make him dentures."

Another villager had an extreme John Gilbert profile and my technician had confessed that if this chap ever lost his teeth his chin would touch his nose. Well he did, and it did. The important point here is that when the teeth are lost the surrounding bone goes too; it resorbs leaving just the basal jaw bones. This can be quite extreme, and trying to fill the gap with dentures was a bit like propping up the roof of the Albert Hall with a four story block of flats. I remember one lady, when asked how her new dentures felt, commented that it felt as though she had a battleship in her mouth.

I cannot recall the final result with these patients but between us I think we got reasonable results. Certainly making the patient happy with the final result is paramount. After all, whenever they walk down the street and smile or grimace at anyone they are advertising your work. It was a steep learning curve for me, those early couple of years, and the technician was a great help in giving snippets of advice on the kind of techniques that were not taught at dental school.

One of the commonest reasons for having to make a new denture, usually in a hurry, is because the patient has lost their beloved prosthesis. The reasons behind the loss can be both tragic and entertaining – usually tragic for the patient and maybe entertaining for the practitioner. In all seriousness there can be an embarrassing gap for the poor unfortunate – not just orally but socially, due to the length it can take to make a new denture. Usually the victim has to hide away in a cupboard for a week while the technician gets bribed to construct a new one as soon as possible. All is not lost (apart from the denture), however, if the patient has a spare set. That got the lady or gentleman out of jail a few times.

The reason behind the loss of a denture is all too often a sorry embarrassing tale, usually involving a degree of over imbibition.

"I lost it speaking to hughey down the big white telephone."

"I wasn't drunk, I'd just had seven vodkas, and then I was sick. It must have been something I ate."

"I couldn't bear to fish it out!"

One poor woman I treated was on holiday in Barcelona with her husband and had climbed to the top of Gaudi's stunning *Sagrada Familia*. As she looked down on the hordes two hundred feet below she exclaimed to her husband "What a wonderful view George...*splut, cough* oh God I've chust yoshed ma wallies." Yes, she watched in horror as her upper denture sailed downwards to crash into a dozen acrylic shards among the astonished Spaniards below. That lady had to postpone her forthcoming retiral party as, even with an understanding technician, I could not make her a new upper denture within ten days.

As you may have gathered many denture losses are down the toilet, although not everyone would freely admit to that. I had one very elegant, urbane lady who returned from her Eastern Mediterranean cruise without her lower denture.

"That's a shame, Mrs Smythe-Parker, how did this unfortunate situation arise?" I enquired delicately.

"I lost them down the toilet while I was being ill after luncheon. The seas were frightfully rough."

In the Aegean? Aye right!

The loss of a denture has produced a good few apocryphal stories about such events – most of them involving rowing-boats and Largs. My favourite is the one about the three fishermen out in Largs Bay on such a craft. Their fishing lines are over the side and eventually Jimmy feels a fish bite. He hauls it upwards and discovers a mackerel struggling at the end of the line. In his excitement to land it his jaws wobble and his lower dentures pops out and disappears into the murky Clyde. His friends, naturally, think this is very funny, and some moments later decide to play a trick on him. Wullie surreptitiously removes his own lower denture, attaches it to his line and lowers it back into the water. After a suitable gap he proclaims he too has got a bite. On reeling in he announces loudly "Jimmy, I've caught yer teeth!"

Jimmy is overjoyed at his good fortune, detaches the denture and proceeds to try it in his mouth. After two fiddly attempts he confesses "Ach, it's no mine," and promptly throws it back into the sea.

Not all such denture disasters are due to losing a denture. Sometimes the denture is simply broken beyond repair. Acrylic is brittle and can break readily, especially if dropped. This often happens while the denture is being cleaned; it simply being dropped into a sink by mistake. Crack! I always advised patients to half fill the sink with water when cleaning them, to cushion any accident.

Dentures were sometimes trodden on - sometimes at home by their loved ones, or occasionally by their beloved dentist. I knew one practitioner who on removing a lady's brand new denture to adjust it accidentally dropped it, then on adjusting his stance, proceeded to step on it and break it in two.

However, and this next bit is a real puzzle, incredibly often the denture was broken into fifty pieces by the family dog! I have no idea why this would happen, perhaps I should ask a vet. Maybe some dogs don't like the arrangement of teeth. Maybe they wanted to try the denture in for themselves. The common denominator was that invariably the denture had been chewed into so many bits that it was rendered into a denture jigsaw.

Repairing a fractured denture usually involves the technician, and he or she is primed to make repairs very quickly so that the patient is inconvenienced for the least amount of time. Normally the patient would appear the next day to collect the repaired denture, and usually, instead of taking up the dentist's time, would be ushered into a private corner of the practice to try the repair in. On one occasion a lady was handed her poly bag containing her denture and instructed to go into the toilet to try it in. Ten minutes passed before she reappeared.

"Is everything okay, Miss Green?"

"No it isn't."

"Does it not fit properly?"

"I don't know yet, I can't get the bag open."

Handing over a repaired denture can create potential problems. I recall on more than one occasion the wrong denture being handed over and a red-faced nurse chasing the patient down the High Street to retrieve it.

Artificial teeth are commonly added to an existing partial denture in situations where the patient needs an extraction but whose denture is otherwise satisfactory. This is known as an 'addition' and is an easy procedure. An impression is taken, instructions given to the technician and the patient reappointed for the following day. At this second visit the offending tooth is removed and the 'added' denture re-fitted. But yes, you've guessed it, sometimes errors can occur here too. You extract the offending tooth and then discover from your receptionist that the denture has not yet returned from the lab. Worse still, you extract the tooth then on refitting the denture find to your horror that the technician has put the wrong tooth onto the plate. One mustn't assume this is the technician's fault here -the wrong instructions may have been issued. These are the kind of things that only happen once, experience learnt from such calamities ensures that in future checks are made before proceeding with the extraction.

I mentioned earlier that I loved denture work. Much of the time I did but there could be challenges. Some patients find wearing a denture next to impossible, but have the ill -advised presence of mind of continuing to try anyhow. There are warning signs.

Mrs Wilson turns up for her first appointment with a polythene bag containing seven sets of full dentures. "I can't really wear any of these."

Meanwhile the dentist is thinking "and you expect me to make you one that's any better?" She then spends the first ten minutes of the valuable appointment time bringing out each set from the bag in turn, and tries unsuccessfully to match an upper with a lower. Spotting clues that would help such a reunion, such as wear on the teeth or the degree of staining, I would try to help.

"It's okay, son, I know my own dentures. Now, this is my first one, oh no this is it, or is it that one."

To add to the confusion she now removes the dentures that are currently inhabiting her mouth and also pops them into the bag.

"Now, you've put me off, where was I?"

Inevitably she then puts the one she has just taken out back in again. Then, realising she is trying to put her lower denture onto her upper gum, flops it out into the bag "That one never fitted right!" And the cycle is repeated. In situations like this the new dentures are never, and I mean never, going to give the patient the result she desires. The dentures in her bag have all been made by different dentists, and in a few weeks' time your new ones are going to join them. Fortunately by then she will be sitting in front of another dentist.

When it comes to picking the shade and shape of the acrylic teeth to put on a new denture it is important that the patient is involved in the process, but it is crucial that it is the dentist who ultimately chooses. Given a Dulux shade card of teeth ranging from snow white to smokers brown the patient will choose the pearliest white shade. This may be fine if the previous denture or natural teeth are similar, and it suits the patient's skin colour. But if the patient is a seventy-eight year old former miner then 'pure dead brilliant white' is probably not the best choice.

Sometimes a patient would prefer to pay privately for their new dentures. This allows a greater range of tooth shape and shade, more technician time and many other features that will cost the dentist more in time and lab costs. Perhaps porcelain, rather than acrylic, teeth will be selected. Porcelain teeth are used less commonly in dentures nowadays and in my experience can be noisy when chewing, and still have a tendency to fall out from the pink gum part of the denture. I remember one old boy who insisted in porcelain teeth in his denture. He was so pleased with them that you could hear them clacking all the way down the High Street in Ardrossan.

Better quality acrylics are usually used in private dentures, but I have to say here, that trying one's best to make a good quality NHS denture was so important. The dentist has to bear in mind that Mrs Brown's new dentures will be displayed to all her regulars at *Morrisons*, the church, the local coffee shop and to all her dozens of friends. In no other branch of dentistry can the dentist really put a blot on their reputation if he or she screws a denture up. Making an adjustment or correction is fine, but it is important to try one's best to get a good result. Most patients realise when you are doing your best to sort out any wee problems that arise and are grateful when you eventually get there.

Occasionally I would visit a patient at home , a domiciliary visit, to attend to their needs when for whatever reason they were not able to come to the practice. It was easy enough to take a tooth out in someone's home, I just brought all the instruments I thought I might need plus a dental nurse. Commonly the domiciliary visits were to construct dentures for an elderly patient, and again this was usually straightforward., but involved four or five visits. When working in Lanarkshire, in the early 80s, an elderly lady, Mrs K, telephoned the practice to ask if a dentist could come out to make her new dentures. I couldn't manage, but a colleague could. He went off to the given address one lunch time, knocked on the door and introduced himself as Mr M. the dentist. After a slight pause he was ushered inside whereupon he examined the patient and suggested to her that she needed new dentures. Over the next four weeks he visited every Tuesday lunchtime, and the dentures were duly fitted. A couple of weeks went by, and the practice received another phone call from Mrs K, asking why the dentist had never come out to see her. It transpired that my colleague had knocked at the wrong door. Strangely, the lady who had opened the door did not think it odd that a dentist would call unannounced, and then proceed to examine her and prescribe treatment! Just as well it wasn't a transplant surgeon knocking the door.

I remember one home visit to a chap's house one lunchtime, to re-cement a front crown that had dislodged. He told me to listen to Saga Radio that evening, as he was being interviewed about some charity work he had done. I did, and there he was, announcing through the ether that the dentist had been out to him that day to "….superglue my front tooth back into my gum." I hope the General Dental Council weren't listening.

Dentures can also be constructed in a metal alloy, usually an alloy of cobalt and chromium, in order to give strength to the prosthesis. Co-Cr alloys are light weight but very strong. Thin bars of this can join the two halves of a lower partial denture or form a neat framework for an upper. Being a denture, these are meant to be removed daily by the patient for cleaning. On one memorable visit to the practice many years ago, however, the down side of this arrangement became odiously apparent. The patient was new to the practice and had been sent along on the recommendation of a good number of his friends, who – well how can I put it – couldn't stand his bad breath any longer. Hints had been flowing in the chap's direction for a number of years until he eventually turned up on my chair. Now dentists are used to smelly breath, it really doesn't bother us, but this was something else. The second he rose up from his seat in the waiting room the remaining patients there started looking at the underside of their shoes. I found it difficult to examine the poor man, for there was a limit to how long I could hold my breath. The cause of the problem was immediately clear, however. He was wearing an upper cobalt-chrome partial denture, which was now – how can I say it without putting you off your tea – somewhat encrusted. Thinking on my feet, some distance from the chair, I prescribed him an antiseptic mouthwash and reappointed him in a week's time. This type of mouthwash is useful as it kills all germs dead – just like a certain well-advertised brand of household bleach. In this case I knew it would chemically clean up his mouth as a temporary solution to his social problem. But before he left I quizzed him about his denture. Did he ever take it out to clean it? Did he have a wife? No he'd never taken it out – he never knew he was supposed to take it out, let alone clean it. How long had he had it? Fifteen years. And no, he was unmarried.

Subsequent visits were much more palatable; I made him a new Co-Cr, and never saw him again. Just as fifteen years were approaching again I decided to retire.

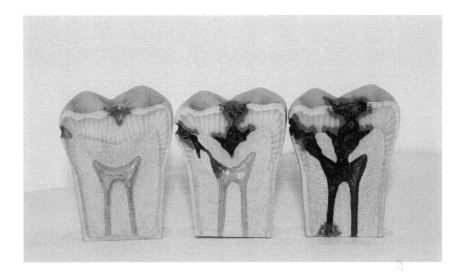

These models give an idea of the progression of dental decay through a molar. On the left there is early decay in the natural grooves of the biting surfaces, with another early spot on the left proximal side. Treatment would be monitoring or simple fillings or sealants.

The middle image shows considerable worsening of tooth destruction with the pulp (nerve) now invaded by decay. This tooth would probably be painful. Treatment would likely involve root-treatment then substantial filling.

The right hand molar shows that the pulp has now died-off, causing an abscess which is spilling out into the surrounding bone. Treatment would have to include root-treatment and filling, or else extraction.

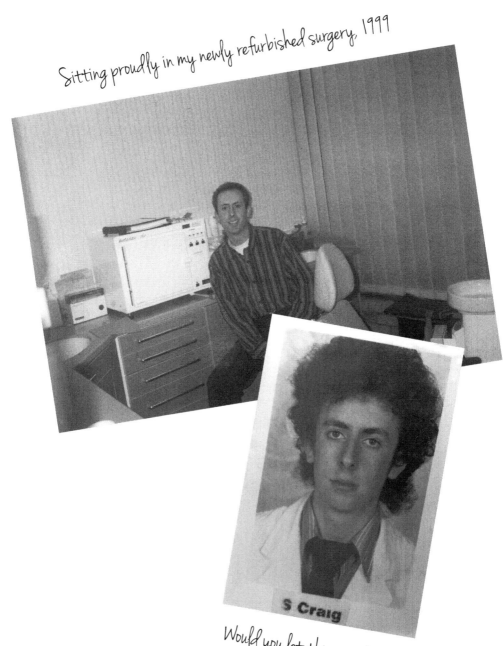

Sitting proudly in my newly refurbished surgery, 1999

S Craig

Would you let this guy loose in
the dental hospital?

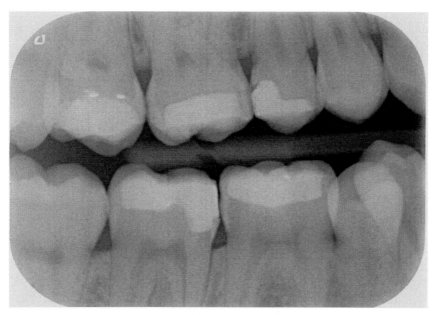

A dental radiograph. The whitened areas are amalgam fillings. There is very early decay at the left hand edge (distal) of the middle tooth on the top. Its neighbour to the right has a gap at the filling, which would need replaced.

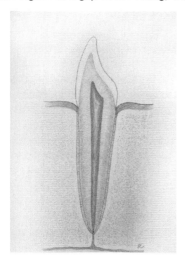

Drawing showing the anatomy of a healthy lower canine.

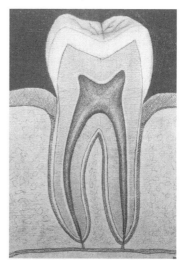

A drawing showing the anatomy of a healthy lower molar.

Gums are important – they hold your teeth in. Quoting the words of the great Tommy Cooper, recalling a visit to the dentist:

"I went to the dentist yesterday, he said my teeth are fine but my gums are going to have to come out."

Never a truer word spoken in jest, I say. More teeth are extracted for gum disease than tooth decay. Basically, poor oral hygiene can cause bacteria to settle deeper into the tissues that support the teeth. Bone is progressively lost and the teeth become gradually, and then dramatically, loose – or as they say in Glasgow *shoogly*.

When a tooth is decayed or otherwise damaged, it can usually be repaired. If it is terminally loose due to gum disease then saving it is much more difficult. So brush those gums, as well as the teeth, and if your dentist has a hygienist visit her, or him, and do as you are told! I don't want to sound severe here, but gums *must* be looked after, by brushing them properly.

The commoner gum disease I referred to earlier is the progressive loss of the tooth supporting tissues due to gingivitis and ultimately periodontitis (inflammation of the deeper supporting tissues). The main cause is poor oral hygiene but there are lots of other factors, including smoking, diet, family history and just bad luck. It can be treated but requires a lot of patient participation to keep it under control. It is generally an unfair world; I've seen many people who hardly ever brush their teeth and gums but had no gum disease. Contrastingly, some poor souls develop an insidious form of chronic periodontitis just by looking at a sweetie! Dentists can prescribe different types of antibiotic, but they are generally of no use in periodontitis, apart from the odd occasion when there is an acute flare-up causing the patient a degree of distress.

One very common, and painful, condition that affects a particular part of gum is *pericoronitis*. This is inflammation under the flap of gum that sits on top of a lower wisdom tooth which has not fully taken up its rightful place at the back of the mouth. It can cause a nasty infection, usually in young adults, and very often antibiotics are needed to shift it. Bear in mind the *wisdom tooth* is not an extra tooth but the normal, third molar which is supposed to erupt at the end of the line to help with our chewing. Often there is no space for them – but that's a long story which I will spare you.

But fear not, for the vast majority of us gum disease, and indeed dental disease in general, is preventable. Trying not to sound repetitious here, but regular brushing with a fluoride toothpaste, and visiting your dentist when summoned are the most important things that are within your control. Brushing properly removes that nasty, sugary, bacterial soup which dental workers call plaque. It is the bugs in the plaque that cause most of the damage. As a rough guide, brushing helps prevent gingivitis and periodontitis, while refraining from sugary snacks and drinks, and the fluoride in toothpaste, prevents tooth decay.

Plaque is the 'baddy'. It teams with bugs – in fact if you could view it under a microscope most of it would be wriggling. Now you wouldn't want that clinging to your teeth and gums, would you?

Flossing is a tremendous adjunct to tooth brushing – if one is motivated to do it. When I first heard of 'flossing', as a lad, I imagined drawing great fluffy clouds of candy floss around the teeth and wondered just how all that sugar would help prevent tooth decay; in fact some people do just that. But floss – the 'thready' stuff – is about the only thing that will get between the teeth and clean away any debris. It takes time and a degree of skill to employ, however.

One fairly new and ingenious way of helping folk brush between their ivories is the use of interdental brushes. These are like miniature bottle-brushes, and are colour-coded to allow the choice of different sizes, depending on the size of the gap between individual teeth. The largest size would be useful on a horse, I suspect. Again, your hygienist is the best person to ask for a demonstration.

Fluoride is an emotive issue, especially when it is voiced that it should be added to drinking water. In my opinion, if people don't want to have fluoride put in their drinking water then they shouldn't be forced to; but if it were there, all it would do is reduce tooth decay. There already are additives in our water, and naturally occurring fluoride minerals exist in much higher amounts than the proposed doses in some parts of the country. Fluoride ions bond readily to tooth enamel and have the effect of strengthening it, making it less vulnerable to acid degradation. So fluoride toothpastes are very important. Other types of toothpaste have come on the market in recent years, for example sodium bicarbonate toothpastes. I am wary of these as they tend to be more abrasive and I have seen significant damage done by over-zealous brushing with them, not just abrasion of the tooth, as mentioned earlier, but stripping of the gingivae around the teeth, causing the soft tissue to migrate away from the tooth and take on a scrubbed, polished look.

"You've been scrubbing your gums again, Mrs Vim, haven't you?"

"Oh no, I've just been doing it exactly as you told me too."

This type of patient will wear the bristles of their toothbrush flat in days. Once a brush loses its shape, has sat on your bathroom cabinet for months or has started to turn green then it is time to invest in a new one. The old one becomes an excellent tool for cleaning the gears on the bike – I can assure you.

It should be obvious that trying not to eat too much sugary crap is the best way of preventing both tooth decay and gum disease. By the way, I never banned sweets among my own children, but snacks were monitored and controlled. We have four children and they never had a decayed tooth between them – it was only their dad who had that, but we won't go into this....nobody's perfect!

The worst kind of sweetie-eating is when sugar snacks are being eaten continuously – one wine gum after another. The mouth is then under constant acid attack from those nasty bacteria and doesn't get a chance to recover. If you must eat a Mars Bar then eat it all in one go, then ideally rinse with water afterwards. You should wait half an hour before brushing, otherwise all that sugary waste will get brushed around the teeth. The same applies to soft drinks loaded with sucrose or glucose. Taking constant sips of these is disastrous.

I knew a sports fanatic who whenever he was at the gym, or out running, constantly sipped a sugary 'health' drink, as it claimed to rehydrate the body effectively. It was also effective at producing holes in his teeth – over a six month period he developed three carious cavities which needed urgent filling. When I explained the cause he was as shocked as I was.

I used to be asked if it was a good idea to use mouthwashes daily. This, yet again, is a personal opinion, but I think antiseptic mouthwashes should be used only when recommended by a dentist or hygienist. There are times when rinsing with chlorhexidine-based mouthwashes is advised by dental professionals. This has excellent antiseptic properties but does stain teeth (temporarily) and should be used only when recommended in certain circumstances, such as a relapse of a periodontal infection. The other weaker antiseptic mouthwashes, of which there is an abundance on supermarket shelves, are fairly useless, in my humble opinion.

Fluoride mouthwashes will strengthen tooth enamel but again I would suggest they are used where the teeth are vulnerable, as recommended by the dentist. Remember, nothing beats thorough brushing with a fluoride toothpaste, for three minutes – while your breakfast egg is boiling. And then maybe brush again after you eat it!

Obviously I am going to say that visiting your dentist for frequent check-ups is crucial. Remember one important point here, your dentist doesn't look at you as a set of teeth walking into his surgery, he or she thinks of you as a person. Your general well-being, or lack of it, is of importance to the dentist. As already mentioned we have been well-educated in general medical stuff and look at the whole person. Many people see their dentist more frequently than their doctor, and so dentists are in pole position to guide you to other medical people if necessary. I've suggested many times to patients who are in for their check-up that they show their doctor that spot on their neck, get the school nurse to give some advice on hair lice, or get their hairdresser to give them a decent haircut.

There has been discussion that visiting the dentist every six months is too frequent. I disagree, six months is ideal, for clearly this can slip. Some people have such a high risk of tooth decay or don't appear to possess a toothbrush, and consequently would benefit from a dental check-up every fortnight. I exaggerate, but you get the picture.

Attending regularly also builds trust and rapport between dentist and patient. Just as the clinician gets to know the patient, and their needs, the person sitting in the dental chair gets to know the dentist. It is a symbiotic relationship and can lead to great understanding between both parties. I was fortunate enough to have treated many great patients – really nice people whom I knew trusted my judgment. With frequent visits the patient often gets into the state of equilibrium where they only need remedial treatment infrequently. You might jump to the wrong conclusion that this doesn't suit the dentist as he/she is not able to provide treatment and thus isn't being paid. But dentists get paid for check-ups, and that wee polish of the teeth. In any case, patients who do not need treatment do not occupy the dental chair for very long. If the nine o' clock patient doesn't need treatment, then no worries, the ten past nine patient will.

Getting the kids into the surgery every six months is crucial to developing their oral health and trust of the dentist. Most parents realise that, and often the visit of a family of youngsters was a real highlight of my day – although, sometimes it was the exact opposite! This becomes somewhat assuaged as time passes when you realise that wee Mary has been visiting you for twenty years and now has a wee Mary of her own – but such is life.

Let me quote from the British Dental Journal of 1895. A dentist identified only as Mr Cunninghame states:

"The great point to be aimed at was to encourage parents to take their children to dentists when the teeth began to decay. If that was done the horrors of the dentist chair would be dispensed with…..I know several cases in which the children had come to look upon a visit at the dentist's with pleasure."

Well, I suppose he should be congratulated for being forward thinking, but I would be tempted to say that children would have spared the 'horrors' better if they had been taken to the dentist *before* the teeth 'began to decay'.

Some of the best inventions in the history of human civilisation came from the Chinese. It is likely that the bristle toothbrush was one of their innovations, dating from around the 15th century. It is a clever invention that has stood the test of time. My advice? Get one and use it! Some people just cannot get the hang of it. I've seen many patients who after being instructed by myself, and then even more brusquely by the hygienist *still* cannot brush their teeth – I'm not talking about 3 year olds here.

"Are you brushing better, Mrs Green?"

"Oh yes, dentist, after getting a row from the hygienist I've really taken it to heart."

I look in her mouth and the plaque is so thick you could plant potatoes around her teeth- which were the same colour as her name.

"Pass me the Massey-Ferguson, nurse, and we'll clean this up!"

One section of society that is generally very good at tooth brushing is young children. A four year old gets very adept at brushing, given proper positive instruction, but then baby teeth are easier to clean. And kids love doing it. They can become so proud of their sparkling little teeth.

By contrast, apparently the Komodo Dragon of Indonesia has the dirtiest, foulest mouth on the planet. The toxins produced by decaying flesh around its teeth mean that one bite can cause death to its victim from blood poisoning. Well, I seek to differ – there's some folk I've had the pleasure of treating…...

Bleeding gums is one of those things that toothpaste companies are always terrifying the life out of you about in their adverts. Gums bleed readily if they are inflamed; and they become inflamed if there is plaque around them. There is no need to panic if a tiny spot of blood hits the sink when brushing, your teeth aren't going to be lying next to you on the pillow the following morning, but it is an indication that you need to be a bit more thorough with that brush. If the sink turns salmon pink then that's a different matter.

When plaque lies against teeth without being removed, either through neglect or difficult access (plaque can lie under the rim of gum) it can harden, or calcify. This chalky deposit is now called calculus and can be very difficult to remove. It's like having hard core on your teeth, although I once described it as such to a gentleman patient and immediately regretted it. Hard, steel instruments are required to chisel calculus off, or else the deployment of the wonderfully effective ultrasonic scaler that dentists and hygienists love. The tip of this instrument vibrates at a very high frequency and with the aid of a jet of water aimed at its tip it blasts plaque and calculus away up the dental nurses' 'sooker' (aspirator). Some patients are not so keen on ultrasonic scalers, as they can be a bit sensitive, but they *do* get the job done. I often wished I could get a shot of it on a Komodo Dragon – provided it was anaesthetised. Some people form huge lumps of calculus over their teeth remarkably quickly and comprehensively. The teeth then look as though they have been plastered over by a trainee builder. Using the ultrasonic on teeth such as these is actually great fun – like power-hosing your patio. Once all the plaque and debris has been blasted away the teeth and gums feel nice: patients generally like the feeling. But within hours a film begins to build up on the surfaces of the teeth again, and this soon becomes colonised with bugs. This is why frequent brushing is essential. It also helps prevent smelly breath, although the causes of this can be complex. So if you find that people are crossing to the other side of the road on your approach then perhaps you're needing to brush a bit better - or wash your armpits.

Now, a word about hygienists. I've worked with several over the years and they've all been excellent. Hygienists are very well trained and skilled in identifying problems with the gums and dealing with them. Once the patient has been examined by the dentist, then often the hygienist takes over to provide any scalings or polishing that is required. They have the time, and all the shiny tools, to remove plaque and calculus from around the teeth, and for most people (except the ones without teeth) regular visits to the dental hygienist will help maintain good healthy gums. The last hygienist I worked with hailed from Nairn, and therefore had a funny accent – to this born and bred *Weegie*. I spent a lot of time popping my head round the door of her surgery and trying to get her to say "Friday" or "seven", which always came out as "Fry-day and Seevan". She soon got wise to me.

"What day are you in next week Ali?"

"The day after Thursday."

"And when are you finishing tonight?"

"An hour after six. Now go away and do something useful."

Hygienists are also great at offering oral hygiene advice, even if it is in a funny accent. They *know* how to keep teeth and gums clean – so listen to them! And can I add at this juncture that I love Nairn and used to go my holidays there.

GETTING TO THE ROOT OF THE PROBLEM

Americans famously call them 'a root canal'. Over on this side of the pond dentists refer to such procedures as 'root-canal treatment'. What does it mean?

All teeth have a soft pulp inside them, running up the root(s) from the bone surrounding the tooth, containing a blood supply and nerve tissue. Without this bundle of soft tissue the tooth would die and indeed would never have developed in the first place. Although securely imprisoned within the roots and pulp chamber of the tooth, this bundle is vulnerable, for its supply line from the rest of the body is narrow, and any trauma or severe movement to the tooth can sever the supply line, leading to the tissue dying off. Trauma includes decay (caries), having the tooth worked on by a dentist or severe traumatic fracture. But dentists can generally fix all these unfortunate misfortunes. This is where root-canal treatment saves the day – and the tooth.

If the pulp tissue – let's call it the 'nerve', for that's what everyone else calls it – dies off, the tooth usually becomes infected inside and this infection can spread into the surrounding bone and soft tissues causing an abscess. This can sometimes be quite spectacular and even life-threatening. It can also be bloody sore. Dentists can treat this by draining the infection (by cutting into the pulp chamber of the tooth to release pressure and infection) and then over a series of visits clean out the root canal and fill it with a bland cement. The tooth can then be refilled or crowned.

Root treatments are fairly easy on front teeth, which normally have just one canal. They become trickier the further back one goes in the mouth. Molars may have three, four or five root canals, and in theory these should all be cleaned out and filled up (obturated) for the treatment to be successful – although this isn't always possible.

Root canals get a bad name. Comedians help perpetuate this with comedic lines such as "I had to kiss my mother-in-law, it was almost as bad as having a root canal!" This reputation that they have acquired is totally unjustified – I loved my mother-in-law. If the nerve has already died out then having a root-canal treatment is usually painless, and often doesn't even need a local anaesthetic. In some situations the tooth is in its last throws of dying and the nerve inside is inflamed. This can be excruciatingly painful and sometimes achieving good local anaesthesia to instigate the treatment can be tricky. But the dentist can usually deal with the problem very quickly. It was one of the pleasures of being a dentist that you could have a patient arrive at the surgery clutching their jaw in agony and have them walk back out fifteen minutes later pain-free and promising you their daughter's hand in marriage.

Most severe toothaches are treated by root-treatment rather than extraction. This wasn't possible until the advent of good local anaesthetics, of which I'll give you another dose later. It is worth explaining just what toothache is, so that if you are ever unfortunate to suffer from it you can understand what the hell is going on.

Toothache can be an excruciating experience for a very good reason. Think of an inflamed spot on your skin. It becomes red and swollen, but is not excruciating because the inflamed tissue can expand. Now, consider the pulp tissue inside, say an incisor. It roughly measures 3mm cubed, but is trapped inside the little chamber inside the tooth; which may turn out to be its coffin. If it becomes inflamed it cannot expand, and this puts a lot of pressure on the nerve fibres in the pulp, which results in pain. Left alone the pulp expands down the root canal to towards the wee hole at the end of the root into which the blood and nerve supply to the tooth comes in from the supporting bone. This expansion eventually puts so much pressure on the pulp tissue that the blood supply cannot get into the tooth and the nerve dies. The tooth is now abscessing, and the pain changes character. Instead of a vague pain the tooth now becomes sore to touch. The pain may now ease as the expanding tissue can reach out into the surrounding tissues. But now you have the risk of infection from the dead pulp tissue. This sequence of events can usually be relieved by root-treatment, and the dentist can usually detect what stage of this pathological pathway the tooth has reached. Identifying the initial cause of pulp pain can be tricky as the pain initially felt from the nerve is often referred to another part of the jaw. For example lower molar pain is often felt in the ear, on the same side. Upper molar pain often radiates to the side of the head. Always on the same side, it never jumps sides. This referred pain is due to the common nerve supply of the teeth as they reach the brain. It can cause real difficulties in diagnosis, but when the tooth starts to abscess then the pain usually becomes more tooth specific. Often a patient attending with vague, intermittent and severe pain on one side would ask if they thought they should be going to the doctor instead of the dentist. That trio of 'vague, intermittent and severe' on one side of the face is classic toothache, from a tooth which is still alive.

Not all toothaches need root-treatment, of course. Sometimes the tooth is sensitive, sometimes a filling is annoying it or the patient may have bit down hard on something they shouldn't have. Usually these teeth can be successfully calmed down by applying medicaments onto the tooth surface or by placing a sedative cement inside the tooth. Often nature will sort out the problem on her own – given a bit of time.

Another very common cause of pain is caused by a crack deep under one of the pointed bits of tooth, called cusps. This usually causes very specific symptoms, which your clever dentist will know all about!

Dentists use a variety of fine instruments to clean out and scrape the root canals, rendering the inside of the tooth squeaky clean. Generally these are divided into two groups: files and reamers. There are more different types of file and reamer than there are stars in the sky. Back in the Dental Hospital days a dozen colour-coded reamers and files of different sizes were laid out neatly, along with lots of other tasty bits and pieces, on the root-canal treatment instrument tray. After the student had finished with the treatment on a given patient, usually about 8.30 at night, these reamers had to be counted to make sure they were all present and correct. One day, one of my colleagues noted that the green reamer was missing. Had it dropped on the floor? Had the patient eaten it? Was it still hanging out of a tooth? When the answer to all these was negative the patient was asked to stand up. No reamer. The tutoring clinician on duty that afternoon had seen this all before, of course, but he always assumed that the only possible answer was that the patient had inhaled it – despite the patient having no recollection of having done so. There was nothing else for it – the patient had to be sent to the X-ray department downstairs for a chest X-ray. Once there the radiographer gave him a white gown and told him to undress completely and don it. He disappeared into a cubicle and emerged four minutes later, wearing the gown and holding a green reamer in his hand. "Is this what you are looking for?" Apparently, and we can only take his word for it, it was trapped in his underpants.

When a patient is about to undergo a root-canal treatment it is imperative that they have an X-ray of the afflicted tooth. The dentist needs to know exactly how long the root is, what shape it is and if there are any pathological issues related to the problem. A second X-ray needs to be taken post-treatment to make sure things are in order. Having a couple of dental radiographs is not a significant risk to the patient as the doze of X-rays is very small and properly filtered; for example a flight to Majorca exposes the passenger to Gamma rays that are equivalent to having two dental radiographs. Patients fully understand this, but an issue may arise if the patient is pregnant and may not want an X-ray taken despite the protective covering that the dentist can offer. In this situation I would explain the low risk to the patient but fully understand if she wanted to abstain. One day, just a few months before I retired, a young woman came in with a painful upper premolar. She was a 'new' patient to the practice. I examined her and diagnosed an abscessing tooth which needed opening up to drain, thus commencing a root-canal treatment. I told her what I was going to do and suggested an immediate radiograph. She hesitated at this point and whispered that she thought she might be pregnant – but wasn't sure as it was 'early days'.

Now there is no problem in opening up a root canal without a radiograph, but clearly I would need one at a subsequent visit. So I opened up the tooth, cleaned out the dead nerve tissue and sealed the tooth in the normal manner. I reappointed her for a week's time and requested that if she had any confirmation of her pregnancy that she could then let me know.

A week later she came in, looking a bit dour but announcing that she was indeed pregnant. I picked up my mirror and probe and started to examine her tooth.

"So last week I opened your tooth to drain." Picking away at the temporary cover I had placed on her premolar at the previous visit I enquired "So has there been any reaction?"

She responded delightfully "I haven't told my mum yet?" Then looking up at me and giggling "Oh, you mean from last week's treatment, don't you?"

At that point we both burst out laughing. I am glad to report that her mum was delighted, she gave birth to a beautiful baby girl and the root treatment was a success.

Less pleasing for the practitioner is dealing with abscessed baby teeth in young children. These teeth cannot be root-canal treated as the roots eventually dissolve away to allow the tooth to exfoliate. So in minors extraction of the infected tooth is the only answer, and in very young children that takes all the patience and decoy techniques that the dentist can summon. It wasn't the actual extraction that caused the grief it was the gentle persuasion required (while holding a syringe behind my back) that the forthcoming episode was in the wee angel's best interests. That could be tough, especially if this little Gabriel had been down this road before.

"I'm not going to hurt you!"

"Aye you are!"

"Just a little scratch."

"Naw it isnae, yer no scratching me, and what's that behind your back?"

Frequently it *was* a wee cherub in the chair, and pangs of guilt would flood over me as I pulled back the cheek to insert a needle into that innocent smiling face hoping, for the sake of all in the room and those within earshot in the waiting room, that the face would still be smiling twenty seconds later. In truth, most children are very brave when it comes to such invasive procedures and once numbed the teeth succumb easily.

Usually I could suss whether wee Mary was going to allow a small injection or not within the first few seconds of her sitting in the chair. The dentist cannot force the child to have the treatment and when they make up their mind this is not for them then it is often the parent who is most disappointed. I've had mum or dad (it's usually mum, as dad tends to shy away from such confrontation) plead, bribe, extort, threaten and scream (always in that order) at their little loved one for an hour to let the nice Mr dentist-man give them a tiny wee jab. Sometimes they yield, often they don't.

The sad and wholly preventable issue here is that the child has the decayed and abscessed tooth in the first place. If the child is stuffed full of sucrose most of the day then the inevitable will ensue, and it will be painful and traumatic for all involved – patient, parent and dentist – from then on.

Having said all that, most children make excellent patients, sometimes it's the adults that scream like a baby.

PUT A CAP ON THAT

Where I come from, Glasgow a dental crown is known as a cap. They are also referred to as 'screw-ins' (not by dentists), but we'll come to that later. A crown is basically a whole artificial tooth fitted over an existing tooth to improve its appearance or restore it functionally. The tooth underneath, which must still have a root, is prepared in a particular fashion and the crown, constructed by a dental technician, very accurately fits over the top and is cemented into place. Sometimes multiple crowns are constructed at the same time, and the result can be a dramatic improvement in the appearance of the mouth in general.

Crowns are usually made of porcelain as this has a very natural appearance. They often have a precious metal core, usually an alloy of palladium, to enhance strength.

If a tooth is missing, the teeth on either side of the gap can be prepared for crowns and a row of these, joined together, is constructed to fit over the prepared teeth and the middle gap. This is a 'bridge' and can save the patient from wearing a denture.

If the tooth to be crowned has been root-treated a metal post is fitted into the root to support the crown. This is called a 'post crown' – but in the West of Scotland often referred to as a 'screw-in'.

Crown and bridge work involves highly skilled work by both dentist and technician, which is why they can be expensive. Back (posterior) teeth can also be crowned, the commonest reason being a molar that has become badly broken down after years of being heavily filled. This is a very good way of restoring teeth which are functionally very important, however the NHS will not usually fund the crowning of back teeth.

When crowning a front tooth it is very important to get the shade of the crown correct – to match the colour or tint of the adjoining teeth. This is the responsibility of the dentist, and to help him/her we have a 'shade guide' representing around twenty shades of white; think of a Dulux paint colour chart, with the only options being different shades of white and you'll get the picture. In good light the dentist chooses the appropriate shade and gives this information to the technician. There can be various different shades within the one tooth. Perhaps yellower near the gum margin and greyer at the biting (incisal) edge. Technicians can put several shades into the one crown however, to achieve a very close match. When the crown returns from the laboratory the dentist checks the shade, removes the temporary crown that has been fitted and cements in the new crown - provided it fits well and the bite is fine. If several crowns are being made at the same time then choosing a shade is usually easier. There are areas of potential trouble here, however.

Years ago I was crowning the front six upper teeth on a middle-aged lady. I decided to split the work into two sessions. I would crown the upper left three first, then return to crown the upper right. The first lot were fitted and the shade I had chosen (B2) looked fine. I then proceeded to work on the second lot, and naturally told the technician to make these B2 as well. Where I failed was in not checking the shade of the first lot once they were in place. Like the batch numbers on wallpaper, there can be subtle differences. Any given shade can vary very subtly from one porcelain mix to another. If I had checked I would have noticed that the first set of crowns were slight whiter, a B 1.5 rather than a true B2. So the second set of crowns arrived and I cemented them in. But this lot were a touch darker than a true B2, say a B2.5. When sitting next to each other in the mouth the disparity was obvious to me, and to the patient too. I had to get a whole new set made – an expensive lesson that I was never to repeat.

It is important never to let the patient choose the shade of their forthcoming crown. Equally important not to show the patient their crown until it is tried in place. When held in the hand, or sitting on the dentist's instrument tray the crown can look awfully dark. It looks its best *in situ*.

Shade guides are an endless focus of fascination for patients. Their comments are predictable:

"Is that a Dulux colour card you have?"

"Can I have the whitest one please?"

"Surely my teeth aren't that dark?"

"I'm afraid they are Mrs Smith, in fact you're off the scale."

The different shades on the guide are grouped into short sets titled A, B, C and D depending on the tints in them. For example C shades are a bit greyish and B shades yellowish. Within each group there are four further shades light to dark. Thus A1 is the whitest, A4 the darkest. One day I was choosing from the A shade range for a young chap's new front crown. My nurse was waiting patiently by my side to note down the shade chosen. I hesitated slightly as I tried to decide between an A2 and an A3.

"Okay, let's see, give me an A.....(pause)."

To our collective astonishment the patient immediately burst into song.

"Ai......!"

He let the note go, looked up and said "I've just done something silly, haven't I?"

This remains one of the funniest moments I've ever had in the surgery.

Crowns can fall out, particularly if they are post crowns. The post that holds the crown to the root canal is subject to a lot of stress when biting or chewing, and the luting cement can give way. These can be re-cemented, provided the patient was able to rescue it when it gave way. On more than one occasion this rescue wasn't possible, and down it went – swallowed. Clearly this is not a desirable situation, and one that may take a day or two to resolve, depending on the speed of its journey. Sometimes the patient would appear sheepishly a couple of days later, holding out a highly polished, gleaming white crown on the palm of their hand.

"Well we'll just stick this back in for you."

Most of the work involved in providing a crown is in the preparation of the host tooth. This has to be trimmed and shaped into a specific shape, allowing for the bite with the opposing tooth and sufficient space for the thickness of the crown material. Impressions are then taken and a shade chosen. The impression materials used when making crowns is a very accurate rubber-based material. It is expensive but records fine detail with great precision – which is what the technician needs when a fraction of a millimetre is critical. As the technician will need a few days to fabricate the crown, a temporary crown then needs to be fitted on the prepared tooth. This can be quite a skilled process, as the patient wouldn't thank you for fitting an outsized tombstone to their front incisor. Temporary crowns are made of a type of plastic which is not only absorbent but has a special affinity to the yellow spice turmeric, commonly found in curries. Most of the time I would remember to point this out to the patient, but sometimes I would forget. In the latter case the patient could turn up the following week with their front tooth the colour of a banana.

There is a balance to be set between providing a good quality temporary crown and providing a superb quality temporary crown. If the temp is *too* good there is always the risk that the temporary looks better than the permanent, porcelain one. Likewise, there is a balance to be struck regarding the fit of the temporary crown. The temp needs to stay in place for a week to ten days, and then be able to be removed by the dentist. A common problem is trying to remove a stubborn temp; this is common where there is a row of crowns being provided at the same time.

Back at the lab, the technician makes casts of the mouth and sections them in a way that will allow him, or her, to craft an individual tooth. On this plaster tooth the crown in built up in wax. This wax pattern is then invested in a special plaster and the wax boiled out. The metal alloy which will form the base of the crown then replaces the space the wax was in. Once cooled this is trimmed and layers of opaque cements and then porcelain are built up, in different shades as already described. The porcelain crown then has to be fired, several times, in an oven and then glazed. Clever, isn't it? Well indeed it is, as I said earlier, technicians are smart people.

One of the most successful cosmetic treatments for improving the appearance of front teeth is the provision of porcelain veneers. These can provide excellent aesthetic results when the incisors are stained or heavily filled or not as prominent as the patient would like. Veneers can be made from composite (white filling) material, but are usually made from porcelain. Much less tooth is removed for veneer preparation compared with crown preparation. Again, the veneer is fabricated by the technician and when it returns from the lab it resembles a finger nail, of porcelain. They are delicate until glued (luted) to the tooth. There are many situations when veneers are not appropriate, for example if the patient has very prominent teeth to begin with, or if their bite (occlusion) is unsuitable. I well remember a certain 'make-over' programme on the telly where patients had various aspects of their physical being – shall we say – upgraded. Their teeth were included in this and the resident dentist was obviously a fan of porcelain veneers, even if, in my humble opinion, some of them were unsuitable candidates. Each episode the victim emerged from the surgery looking like the brighter half of a piano keyboard.

Another very successful way of improving the patients' smile is by tooth whitening. This is covered in a later chapter.

A BAG OF NERVES

The witty American poet Ogden Nash once wrote: "there is physical fear and psychological fear. But there is one fear that is both – dentistry." He was being very unkind to dentists here, but then he wrote that a few decades ago. Let's face it, even as late as the 1950s and 60s most dental procedures were not exactly a bundle of laughs, apart from the 'gas' days. Young people, and the not so young now, have no recollection of that as dentistry has improved so much. With no prejudices they trot along to the dentist with no fears and positively enjoy a little pampering from the health care professionals. Great, isn't it?

A few older people who were around before these enlightened times have genuine fear, indeed sometimes phobia, of visiting the dentist. I found these people could almost invariably be 'brought around' with simple, reassuring communication and delicate treatment regimes. Basically just a little TLC, which all dentists should be able to deliver. I've seen patients who were clearly terrified becoming relaxed, keen patients within just a couple of visits. My advice to any nervous patient is to find a dentist whom they can communicate with and to attend regularly.

I have an understanding of phobic patients – for I was once one myself - no really I was. Our family dentist was in Govan in Glasgow's south side. He was a very nice man, but he didn't believe in saving deciduous teeth if there was the slightest excuse for whipping them out. My recollection of visiting the dentist in the 1960s was having a quick check-up and then being given an appointment for the following Saturday for an extraction – under general anaesthetic. I don't remember ever being in pain, but if there was a hole in the tooth - or perhaps just a wee stain - it was coming out; and one of my lower permanent molars went the same away.

So I would turn up that next Saturday, starved, pale and feeling, frankly, terrified; looking, in fact, like what could reasonably be described as 'a contraindication for a general anaesthetic'. My Dad was always the parent who drew the short straw and accompanied me. In those days my dad didn't have a car, so a visit to the dentist involved a bus journey and then a trolley-bus journey. When I saw one of these silent killers purring along with their strange hum, rear double axles and long spidery roof poles a feeling of mild panic would envelope me, for whenever I was on a trolley-bus I was going to the dentist. I was delighted when they left Glasgow's streets for good.

Parked across the road from the surgery was an alternative mode of transport - the anaesthetist's car. It was always a fancy sporty one, and suitably coloured blood red.

I remember the walk up to the door, Dad ringing the doorbell, and Jean, the ubiquitous receptionist, opening the door with a disguised smile. The waiting room would be packed with grim-faced lambs to the slaughter.

Looking out through the corrugated, frosted windows the passing traffic looked distorted and elongated. I wanted to be somewhere else – anywhere.

My name would be called and I would look around, hoping that there was another, more deserving, Stuart in the room. Alas no, was ushered into an ante-room where three seats were positioned in front of a huge porcelain sink. After a visit to the toilet I was told to sit there; my dad now left in the waiting room. Suddenly the door of the surgery would open and a patient would appear, propped up on either side by dental nurses. He or she would stagger to the sink in front of me and proceed to spit out copious amounts of blood. Face wiped they would then be helped out into the hallway, at which point one of the nurses would smile at me and say "are you next?" I went through this ordeal about five times in my boyhood. Now do you understand why I was a dental phobic? Strangely when it was my turn to stagger to the sink, some ten minutes later I always felt pharmacologically euphoric. There I was, staggering out like a baby giraffe, high-stepping out of the surgery over an imaginary threshold.

When I was about six, my big brother – who was then about 18 - had all his remaining teeth extracted and full dentures fitted. I can remember him returning from that Saturday morning surgery and being practically carried upstairs. At my tender age I naturally assumed that this was a fate that awaited me in a dozen years' time.

Up until I was fifteen I dreaded my mum telling me that she had made my routine appointment. Then things changed for the better. The trolley buses had gone and a new dentist appeared at the practice. He was young, chatty, and gentle, and he believed that teeth could be restored. I needed teeth removed for orthodontic reasons and this turned out to be a painless experience. I never again had the terror of a visit to the dentist, although to this day I'd still rather go to *Ikea*. Interestingly, that young dentist who changed my perception of dentistry went on to become dean of Glasgow Dental Hospital.

During my visits to the Dental Hospital (for my ortho treatment) I became interested in what was going on around me. That interest became sustained and soon became a fascination. I found a textbook in my local library on dental pathology and, although I couldn't make head nor tail of most of it, my interest developed and soon I was telling my astonished parents that.... one day I was going to be a dentist. My Mum laughed!

Returning to the 'gas man'. General anaesthetics are no longer performed in general dental practices, and indeed no longer at Glasgow Dental Hospital either. This is clearly a good thing. General anaesthesia is safe, but must be administered under proper clinical conditions. Many poor souls died in the dental chair from reactions to anaesthetics, often they were children; what tragedies.

Dentists themselves used to be allowed to administer the anaesthetic but this was dying out by the time I entered dentistry. I did, however, as a student perform extractions under GA at the dental hospital, with the anaesthetist calling sharply in my ear to get a move on! Thankfully these days have also gone.

Coming back to my own dentist. He practised in a time when removing a decayed deciduous tooth seemed the easiest and best option. Perhaps during his training he had read this extract, from the British Dental Journal of 1894, quoting Mr Edmund Owen FRCS:

"While he would not for a moment suggest that carious (decayed) milk teeth should never be conservatively treated (filled) he, at the same time, thought that this treatment was carried too far." The words in brackets are mine. Thank goodness attitudes from dental workers have changed, although in the same pages of that journal another dentist observes that "... parents very seldom brought their children to the dentist until they suffered pain, and then it was too late to do very much." This is less common nowadays as the attitude of most parents has changed as well. I can think of fewer worse situations, for all involved, than bringing a nervous child to the dentist in pain, when they have never been to a dentist before in their short lives. Believe me, I had to deal with this kind of situation many times.

I obviously do remember some very nervous patients that just couldn't help their disposition. Most of us can get nervous about something. I always have a bubble in my tummy whenever I find myself in an airport – even if I am not flying! But the important issue, as I see it, is that 'nerves' can be conditioned and controlled. Some unfortunates don't seem to be able to do either, however, when they visit a dentist. I can remember a lady who shook so much that I had to hold her jaw still – and that was just when she was talking to me. A common manifestation of nerves is when a patient sits on the chair and keeps one foot on the ground, as if ready to make a run for it if their predicament were to take a turn for the worse. In all my years I only recall one chap doing just that – running out the door, that is. It can work the other way, I have often felt like putting my coat on and running out the door too.

Occasionally nerves take over to the extent that routine actions such as merely getting onto the dental chair are compromised. One morning, when I was working in Lanarkshire, I greeted a patient at the surgery door and in my usual, reassuring way asked her to take a seat. Instead of perching herself on the dental chair she chose, perhaps wisely, the little chair in the corner of the room, as far away from me as possible. On another occasion, again in Lanarkshire, I motioned to a middle-aged lady to sit in the chair. I turned to open my notes and on spinning back round found the lady sitting on the chair, legs apart on either side, facing the wrong way. My nurse had to leave the room, while I struggled to keep a straight face and gently suggested that it might be more comfortable if she was to face the other way. Perhaps she thought she was having a check-up at her gynaecologist.

Very apprehensive patients are sometimes eligible for a course of hypnotherapy to help them get over their fears. This can be very effective, but patients have to be chosen carefully. I recall a chap that was sent to a dental hypnotherapy expert to try to get him to stop biting his cheek, a habit he had got into awhile back but which was beginning to make the inside of his cheeks look like pink loofahs. He returned to the surgery some weeks later to tell me about his experience. The hypnotherapist had used a common trick: getting the relaxed subject to gently raise an arm before proceeding to phase two - pushing a sharp medical needle through the fold of skin between thumb and forefinger.

"I felt so relaxed," he told me. "When he passed the needle through my hand the result was remarkable."

"Really! Was it painless?" I asked.

"Painless? I nearly went through the roof!"

Don't let this put you off - hypnotherapy has a place in dentistry, and as an undergraduate I performed a fair bit of it myself. It didn't work trying to get a dental nurse to go out with me, but it certainly calmed a few patients down.

As I said earlier, we all need a dentist at some point in our lives - just as we all need people from all walks of life; such is the society we find ourselves in. We even need bank managers - do we? Yes, I suppose we do. I certainly needed a few when I was setting up my own practice. I had drawn up cash-flow sheets and, as *Dragons' Den* hadn't been invented, had gone along, cap in hand, and chapped on the door of our friendly, neighbourly Mr Bank of Scotland. He gave me what I wanted, but as someone wiser than me once said, 'a bank lends you an umbrella when the sun is shining, but wants it back as soon as it starts to rain'. Well, after a few months, when business wasn't blooming as I had envisaged, the clouds started to gather, and it poured. Mr Bank gave me a hard time of it. I had fortnightly meetings, or should I say confrontations, with him, and I would trip along to these feeling like....well, like someone going to the dentist. I was nervous, and it showed. He seemed to love it, and bluntly pointed out that I had no money, but I could hold on to the umbrella a little longer. But things turned around, I merged practice with my good pal and soon the sun was shining again. I moved business premises, and lo-and-behold who should come in one day but dear old Mr Bank. He had toothache. I saw him and immediately noted his nervous discomfiture. The umbrella was now truly in my hands, in the shape of a set of forceps. In truth we could both see the funny side of this and we got on just fine. On his way out of the door he turned to me and asked "what do you do with all your money?"

Some people whom you wouldn't necessarily expect to be nervous patients were near wrecks when they attended, for even a routine check-up. One lady who frequently appeared in that state was a policewoman. She often attended in uniform; it was strange to see a police officer looking so worried and pale, but she explained that she would rather face a man with a knife than a dentist with a mouth mirror. I met her by chance in Paisley once, again she was in uniform. As I stopped to say hallo she froze, grabbed her colleague's arm and stuttered "oh my God, it's my dentist!"

"It's alright, I'm unarmed," I replied.

It is an interesting point, that in the surgery, as well as out on the street, the dentist can spot the nervous patient immediately, no matter how they try to hide it. I fully understood how they felt, as I was more than capable of exhibiting the same signs, given the right situation.

Of course the dentist can get nervous too, especially if things aren't going well. My worst nightmare was trying to fit a bridge that clearly wasn't going to. It would be an inconvenience to all concerned if it had to be re-made, but nerve racking the second time around if it still didn't fit, even if I tried to fit it by turning it upside down and inside out.

I used to get very anxious about a particular lady whose visits I dreaded. It seemed that everything I did for her went wrong – and yet she kept on coming back. Frequently I would even get her name wrong, which immediately got things off to a bad start. I wanted to tell her that there was an excellent dentist just down the road! But no, she would turn up to terrorise me on a regular basis. The girls got wise to this, and would wind me up. Just before we finished up on a Friday before a Bank Holiday weekend one would pop her head around the door and say "have a nice weekend. Do you know Mrs Frump's coming in at nine on Tuesday?"

Nurses rarely got nervous. They could handle it all, usually in a very professional manner, even when wee Jimmy was sick and the dentist hurriedly left the room, with the tacit nod that meant "Come and get me when it's all over." I kid not, there were some things that I couldn't stomach, and a patient being sick was one of them. Fortunately it was an extremely rare occurrence. The worst case was when one morning a young woman filled the wee chairside bowl (spittoon) with her partially digested breakfast. I refer to this third hand because I had left the room some seconds previously, and my very capable nurse found me cowering behind a filing cabinet some minutes later.

Rarely did a dental nurse upset the apple-cart and put the patient into a worse state than they were before they entered. I can think of one notable exception. One thing I wouldn't tolerate was a nurse whispering to me or a colleague in front of a patient. The only exception to this was when she wanted to intimate that my favourite mid-morning chocolate bar had arrived in the staff room. If a patient hears whispers they inevitably think we're whispering about them, and this unnerves them, understandably. Brenda was quite a new nurse to the practice. She was aspirating (sooking up) while I was using the ultrasonic scaler to clean a chap's teeth. She kept whispering a series of questions to me - fair enough, I love being asked questions, but not whispered.

Once the patient had left I said to her "Brenda I am happy to answer your questions but please don't whisper, just come out and ask."

In came the next patient - another scaling. A couple of minutes into the procedure I could see Brenda straightening herself - another question was coming. This time, in a loud voice "Where's all that blood coming from?"

THE GOOD OLD DAYS

I am never sure which era old folk are referring to when they talk about 'the Good Old Days'. As I mentioned earlier, being a dental patient when there were refined sugars around, but no anaesthetics to relieve the agony of having teeth yanked out couldn't have been a pick-n-mix of laughs.

History is sprinkled with gruesome, gory stories of toothache and dental surgery. Rabbie Burns even wrote a poem in 1786, *Address to the Toothache*, dedicated to the misery it caused. It wasn't just the proletariat that suffered. King Henry Vlll was alleged to have had a smelly mouthful of abscesses – no wonder he kept having to re-marry. His daughter, Queen Elizabeth l, apparently spent much of December 1578 suffering from toothache. A tooth could always be pulled out, of course, usually by the blacksmith, local doctor or barber, that wasn't the issue. The issue was - which option is the least worse? Having the toothache or suffering the agony of having it removed. As for root-treatments, well let's not go there. Okay, just for a short while then: nowadays inflamed pulp tissue can be numbed and painlessly removed, as described in a previous chapter. In the 'Good Old Days' a miniature red hot poker would be pushed into the pulp. Ouch!

The world was just crying out for dentists to be invented. And in the 18th century they final were – and the world has been smiling ever since! One of the people who deserves a big pat on the back is dentist Horace Wells, from Connecticut in the USA. In December 1844 Horace attended a demonstration on the effects of 'laughing gas' (nitrous oxide or N2O to those of you who passed your chemistry O-grade) when inhaled socially. This gas had been first prepared some seventy-two years earlier, but it was good old Horace that realised this intoxicating vapour could have medical uses; and he tried it out on himself the next day, allowing his colleague to extract a tooth. From then on nitrous oxide was used to anaesthetise patients during surgical procedures. It is still in use today, indeed is the active ingredient in the 'gas and air' mix sucked in by mothers-to-be in the delivery room. In fact, years ago, the then 'father-to be' writing this can attest to its relaxing qualities, during the stress of impending fatherhood.

Poor Dr Wells did not have a life as happy as his gas, sadly. He became addicted to that other powerful knock-out agent chloroform, which clearly altered his judgement. In a prison cell accused of attacking two prostitutes he committed suicide by cutting along a major leg artery – not before anesthetising himself first, of course –using chloroform.

The development of anaesthetic agents allowed the advancement of surgical techniques, both general surgery and dental surgery. There are two kinds of anaesthetic – general and local. The former puts you to sleep, the latter numbs the area to be worked on. Nowadays an intra-venous injection knocks you out, and then anaesthesia is maintained by nitrous oxide or halothane gas.

The first anaesthetic agents were ether and chloroform. These are not used nowadays as they are less safe that nitrous oxide. For one thing ether is very flammable and there are reports in the dental press of explosions occurring in surgeries during dental operations. Indeed the 1925 Journal of the American Medical Association of Anaesthesia relates the tragic case of a poor 16 year old lad undergoing surgery for a fractured jaw sustained while riding his bike. He was given ether and oxygen. Suddenly, when the surgeon was drying the lad's mouth with warm air, there was an explosion at the back of the mouth. The poor chap was dead within ten minutes. This was by no means uncommon. In 1937 the American Society of Anaesthesiologists reported 230 similar explosions, which sadly resulted in 36 deaths and 89 injuries. One explosion in an operating theatre resulted in all the surgeons and nurses being blown onto their backs – the patient survived.

Local anaesthetics are much easier to use and incredibly safe drugs, nowadays! The first 'local' to be used pharmacologically was cocaine, followed by procaine (novacaine) and now superseded by excellent agents such as mepivacaine, lignocaine and prilocaine. Injected over a nerve, or into the tissues surrounding a tooth, they are incredibly effective at stopping nerves from firing, thus preventing pain. However, just as there were some tragic deaths from general anaesthetics, then so there were a few from the dangerous cocaine also.

An early edition (1899) of the British Dental Journal (BDJ) relates an incident where a female patient collapsed after the topical administering of cocaine on cotton wool pellets, being used to make the patient's gum numb. No injection – just dabbing the stuff onto the gum. The lady recovered.

Not so lucky was Lizzie Hamill. The same journal of 1918 related the sad case of this thirty-four year old lady. She was receiving treatment from an 'unqualified practitioner of dentistry' Mr Alexander Scotland. At the inquest Lizzie's sister described how, from the adjoining room, she heard her sister in the surgery moaning. The dentist thumped his foot on the floor to summon help from his son downstairs. Eventually a nurse called the sister into the surgery, and there was poor Lizzie slumped in the chair. The sister, suspecting all was not well, called "Oh Lizzie, Lizzie, are your dead?"

Presumably she never got an answer, for Lizzie was. But Lizzie did not die from a general anaesthetic, but from the administration of cocaine. Powerful stuff, eh?

Dentists were well aware of the dangers that anaesthetics posed, in terms of their volatility and their potent pharmacological effects. Some of the practitioners of the drugs were none too popular either. In his 1916 book

The Manual of Surgical Anaesthetics H B Gardner writes:
"...many a dentist has suffered great inconvenience from the type of anaesthetist who blows up the gas bag with a roar, asphyxiates the patient and then walks unconcernedly away leaving the dentist struggling with a violently jactitating patient." (Yes, I had to 'look up' jactitating as well.)

A coroner looking into the death of Annie Thompson in 1918 gave his verdict that the patient had died during the administration of 'the usual anaesthetic' – cocaine, and although he concluded that there was '...nothing improper in its administration' and that the operator '...did all that was possible' he did feel that 'anaesthetics should be administered by a qualified person.' I think most of us would agree with that.

Mr W McGregor Young MB MS, writing in the BDJ of 1900 would probably have agreed but seems confident enough in the anaesthetic agents around at the time to mix them into a powerful cocktail. He favoured Schleich's Mixture, which he formulates as being "1 part chloroform, 4 parts sulphuric ether and ½ part petroleum ether". Enough to knock out a horse, I wonder. But Mr Young feels that ".....in competent hands is perfectly safe." However in cases of collapse he advises the operator to give a "...hypodermic injection of strychnia." As you may guess from the name, strychnia is derived from strychnine, which is a highly toxic alkaloid, derived from a plant, and used as a rat poison, or sometimes by nefarious wives as a husband poison. Strychnia was used in medicine as a nervous system stimulant. You can see that a hundred years ago dentists had whole cabinets full of dangerous drugs and remedies, and were not shy in using them.

It wasn't just the drugs that could be lethal. On ploughing through the dental literature I found an example of an inquest into the death of a seven year old boy in South Shields. He had died of sepsis from his decayed teeth. Please be reassured that such things don't happen anymore. Today we live in 'The Good Olde Days' of safe modern medicine, and dentistry - be rest assured. Now that general anaesthesia is confined to hospitals and only performed by the big boys, and girls, dentistry has become incredibly safe. In all my 33 years in practice we rolled out the oxygen cylinder just once; we had to blow the dust off it first, before trying to remember how to turn it on. This was just to help a wee old lady recover from a faint. When she returned for her next appointment a couple of days later we had it hidden behind the chair - just in case.

Maybe we were just lucky in not experiencing any medical emergencies. Aside from the wee lady above, faints are common in dental clinics, and are easily managed – as long as it's not the dentist!

Patients are more likely to feel odd if they are in a strange environment, where they don't know anyone. In general practice, where usually the dentist and patient and nurse all knew each other well, faints were less common, in my experience. I had one smashing patient who I did mountains of work on: crowns, bridges, fillings, root treatments, the whole dental pharmacopeia. And she was a very relaxed, delightful patient. But on the rare occasion when I had to extract a tooth she would faint. She forewarned me about this trait whenever I first met her. I think I had to do a couple of extractions over a five year period, and on those occasions we brought her in as the last patient of the day, took her tooth out and then laid her horizontally on a small couch for ten minutes. Then she was fine.

Another way of avoiding faints is to treat susceptible patients later in the day – after they've had their lunch. Many of us are not at our best first thing in the morning. One chap really took us all by surprise, however. It was a tricky extraction but he kept reassuring me he was fine. Job done, he sat up in the chair, gave a bloody smile and conked out. It was so sudden. We put the chair back "Can you hear me, Mr Vagal?" It was a very long twenty seconds before he could. When he came round

he was very confused – he thought he was in Benidorm, and that the dental nurse was his wife.

The only other faint I recall being a bit concerned about was an eight-month pregnant woman, on whom I was doing some treatment which I really ought to have postponed. She felt faint, we put her back on the chair and she felt better. Then she got a pain low down in her tummy. For a few worried seconds I thought we were going to have to get her to sit the other way round in the chair and deliver her baby.

Returning briefly to the subject of general anaesthesia: during my career I had at least a dozen, older patients, who on explaining the filling or extraction I was about to do would then settle down into the chair, and ask if I was going to put them to sleep. I reassured them that had that been the case they would have been forewarned, and that we didn't 'do' that anymore. To which my nurse would add "it's just his chat that will put you to sleep!"

Dental health has clearly improved dramatically over the last sixty years, since NHS dentistry came into being. Despite all the good work dentists and hygienists do, the main reason for the turnaround is dental health education. Everyone is now taught about good oral hygiene and how to keep their mouths clean. They should also know that sugar is bad for the teeth. People are interested in their oral health now, just as they are about their general health – well most people. The dental profession must take a fair amount of credit too – but then I would say that. The 'Good Old Days' are behind us – welcome to a bright, smiling future.

WHITER THAN WHITE

"Does he do cosmetic dentistry?" Our receptionist would often be asked.

The answer is quite straightforward: all dentists *do* cosmetic dentistry. If placing a white filling in a front tooth isn't cosmetic, then what is? Of course, the caller's question refers to a deeper meaning of the term, but the answer is still the same. Dentists are experts at matching the shape, contour and colour of anything artificial that they are placing in someone's mouth.

Years ago I read a joke in a dental journal which went something like this - patient: "can you suggest anything for yellow teeth?"

Dentist: " How about a brown tie?"

Times have changed and there are more treatment options now. Tooth-whitening is all the rage nowadays, and I did a fair bit of it - to my patients, that is, not myself. The procedure is simple: impressions are taken, thin bleaching trays are constructed and the patient supplied with the dental equivalent of *Domestos*. I joke - the whitening agent is usually a compound called carbamide peroxide, but it is a mild bleach. It is very safe, but can cause temporary tooth sensitivity and some gum irritation (while it is being used). These materials can produce excellent results, and without destroying any tooth tissue in the process. Again, like all treatments, cosmetic or otherwise, patients must be chosen carefully, for tooth whitening is most definitely a *treatment* and not a beauty therapy.

In most people tooth whitening works well, but I would always advise people to get their dentist to provide the treatment, and not the wee lassie standing at the corner of Buchanan Street; although regulations on its provision have been tightened recently. My personal reservation about tooth-whitening is that some folk have gone too far. How often do we now get an opalescent, titanium white smile from the guy or gal behind the counter at ASDA or in our local pub? Having spent most of my career providing dentures that were not too white and 'looked natural' I find it rather odd that we now see rows of grinning teeth that look as if they have just been varnished with *Tippex*. I think a lot of the results look very unnatural, but then maybe I am just being old fashioned. I think tooth-whitening looks best if done with subtlety, and if the right subjects are chosen.

I can think of a sixteen year old pleading with me to whiten her teeth, when they were already *Daz* white. I refused. I also refused a fascinating chap who attended me regularly. He wanted his teeth whitened but I refused to do it on the grounds that I didn't think he would benefit from it. You see, he was born in Nigeria. Amos' broad smile always sparkled, and now he wanted to have a whiter sparkle. When checking the shade of his teeth I could see they were of normal shade, but against his black skin they looked beautifully white. The colour of teeth, you see, is influenced by factors around them. How much tooth does the patient show when talking, smiling, laughing? Do they wear lipstick? Yeh, guys wear lipstick too. What tone of skin do they have? I persuaded Amos to spend his hard-earned cash on something else.

Skin colour has to be taken into account in many aspects of cosmetic dentistry. Imagine a row of perfect, pearly white crowns in the mouth of a seventy year old farmer, who has a ruddy, weathered complexion and you get the picture. However, the same shade of crowns would look lovely in the delicate mouth of a pale-complexioned thirty year old. Nowadays assessing skin colour is more problematic due to the fake tan that lots of girls, and as many boys, now don. I can recall picking up a tissue, at the end of a treatment, and wiping the spray from the high speed drill from the tangerine face of a teenage girl. Out of the corner of my eye I spotted my nurse was looking at me and subtly shaking her head. I couldn't see anything wrong with what I was doing and carried on. When I looked at the tissue and saw that it had turned orange I realised I had wiped off a fair percentage of her fake tan. She now looked like a giraffe.

Some denture wearers want whiter than white too. Sometimes I would try to suggest toning them down a bit – but if that's what they really wanted who was I to disagree. I once made full dentures, privately, for three sisters from California who were over in Scotland for the summer. They all wanted the same shade of sparkly, A1 white – and that's what they got. I can remember their departing words before they headed off home "if these teeth are no use we'll come back and haunt you." Scary stuff, but I have yet to be visited by their toothy, spiritual embodiment in the dead of night.

Botox and collagen fillers are also very popular nowadays. I never practised either technique, so I am not going to say anything about it, except that I now see lots of young girls who already had beautiful faces but who now have adopted the look of a trout, with puffy cheeks, a frozen forehead and iceberg teeth. Add in the Groucho Marx eyebrows and the simian look is almost complete. You may gather here that I am not a fan.

Tooth jewellery was in vogue for a while. I had one patient who wanted a zirconium 'pretend diamond' inserted into a tooth, to give him a flashy smile, presumably. I refused. Instead I related to him the story of certain rock band lead man who had an emerald placed into a pre-drilled cavity on a front incisor. He had it removed not long after because he was fed up with people telling him he had a bit of lettuce stuck between his teeth.

Gold fillings at the front of the mouth are different, for gold alloys were used as actual fillings in front and back teeth for many years before the development of white filling materials. These gold inlays were fabricated in wax and cast in high-carat gold alloys. They were then cemented into the cavity. I made many of these, usually at the patient's request until they too went out of fashion. I also made them for acrylic teeth on dentures, again because the patients asked for it, to make the denture look more realistic!

Implants have revolutionised dentistry in recent times, and no wonder. Where a bridge is impossible or destructive to make, and when the patient is not keen on wearing a denture, implants can sometimes be the ideal choice. They have been around for years, but only in the last twenty years have they become much more successful. This is because some clever person discovered that if the implants are made out of titanium instead of steel then they are much more successful. Although not occurring naturally in the body titanium, exhibits an unusual property when used as an implant, whether as a dental implant or as a joint replacement. This strong, dull, brownish metal (have a look at the roof of the IMAX cinema in Glasgow – it's covered in it) is the most biocompatible of metals, in that once placed in bone the body does not reject it and, in fact, goes further by bonding to the surface of the titanium implant in a phenomenon known as osseointegration. This prevents degradation by the body's fluids and leads to strong, non-corroding implants.

Dental implants are screwed into the jaw bone in areas where teeth are missing and then used to hold a frame to support a denture or a bridge. Placed properly by skilled dentists who specialise in this branch of dentistry they are very successful, but expensive. Implants can be used to replace a single tooth, and they can support full upper and lower bridges or dentures. To support a full row of teeth would probably require four to six implants.

I never used implants myself, but often referred patients to those who did. When patients queried the cost I used to compare the expense with buying a car. Cars depreciate the moment you leave the showroom, but implants are likely to give many years of function that could not be achieved by any other dental prosthesis, so they are often worth considering.

Patient attitude towards treatment obviously varies hugely. Some people are extremely fussy about the appearance of their teeth, and the rest of their personage presumably. I suppose there's nothing wrong with that – they keep many dentists in business. Narcissism can catch the dental practitioner out, however. I've handed a mirror to urbane, immaculately turned out professionals, having just completed some front fillings with fifty shades of white employed, all carefully blended, contoured and polished, only for them to take the most cursory of glances and nod in mild appreciation, and then hand the mirror back. In situations like that they would sometimes look at the wrong tooth. "Oh that looks so much better, thank you."

"Actually, it was the one on the other side I just filled."

Conversely, I've employed the same approach to shabby, grey joggy-bottomed, dilapidated souls, only for them to draw the mirror up to their nose and spend five minutes picking holes in my methodology.

"Can you not get that teeth (sic) to match the same colours as the others?"

One lady sat and stared myopically at her restored incisors for ten minutes longer than it took to fill them. I began to wonder if she was actually looking at her teeth at all, perhaps she was having a bad hair day.

"Everything all right?"

"Oh yes, I was just thinking. Who does your teeth?"

A partner or friend in the waiting room can often come to the rescue in situations like these. In cases where the patient was unconvinced about the cosmetic compatibility of my work I often suggested whoever they brought to the practice with them might step into the surgery and provide reassurance. I would then step outside, and either sip a tea or head off home for a nap, depending on how familiar I was with the time my fastidious patient would require. Usually, however, the friend in the waiting room came down on my side.

"Oh that's lovely, Betty, what I lovely job he's made of that."

At this point I would usually hug the friend, and then surreptitiously slip them the promised tenner.

This tactic was not without risks, of course. Had the friend given a contrary opinion I think I would just have reached for my coat and gone off to reconsider my career. It *did* happen once. The 'friend' took one look at the end result and sighed "Oh no, I don't like that at all!"

Bringing friends or relations into the surgery is perfectly acceptable, of course, if that is what the patient wants. When one lady wanted to bring her husband in, as an emotional crutch, while I extracted several of her teeth it somewhat backfired. I had warned against it, but no, she wanted him there. During the avulsion of tooth number three he exhibited all the signs of imminent syncope – he passed out! Like a similar scene from *Fawlty Towers* we had two patients who had to be carried out of the room.

My favourite story about partners being brought into a consultation has nothing to do with dentistry but is worth including here because it is completely true. It was related to me by a doctor friend who was a skin specialist at a well-known Edinburgh hospital. Mr Campbell (we'll call him) was having trouble with a rash on his thighs. The doctor popped out to the waiting room and called gently "Mr Campbell?"

A gentleman, and the lady sitting beside him, rose. They were ushered into the consulting room and sat down opposite the doctor. After a few questions, it was indicated to Mr Campbell that he should remove his trousers and sit on the couch. He did this, and a few more intimate questions were asked.

At this point, his lady companion stood up and asked "Do you think I am with him?"

It turned out that she too was a Campbell, but bore no relation to the patient. She had assumed that patients were being called in two at a time, and the doctor – well he had made a terrible assumption that they were man and wife.

THE PERIODIC TABLE OF DENTISTRY

Prospective dental students cannot get a place in dental school unless they know their chemistry – and the chemistry of everything else around them too. It is studied during the first year of university dental and medical courses, for it is essential to understand chemistry before engaging biochemistry. Without biochemistry the sciences of physiology and pharmacology would be unfathomable. And without those it wouldn't be safe to practise dentistry.

I loved chemistry at school. The labs were a flaunt of capricious black magic, only with logic, and the odd explosion. At school I had six years of it and took it in my stride; organic chemistry was easy at school, but at University it ran benzene rings round me. The chemistry course in first year was tough - an intense lecture every day, with demanding labs and tutorials - but I emerged unscathed, like an irrepressible catalyst at the end of it. So in honour of the enigmatic science of chemistry I dedicate this chapter to the amazing elements that are in everyday use in the art and science of dentistry.

Obviously the human body is constructed using the organic building blocks of carbon, oxygen, hydrogen, nitrogen, phosphorus, chlorine, sulphur, calcium, sodium and potassium, and a few others I cannot remember. Some of the materials used to fill teeth or construct crowns and dentures also contain these elements, but many more are in use.

Amalgam fillings contain silver, tin, copper and zinc in various combinations, and, of course, are mixed with mercury. White fillings are a conglomeration of many elements, including silicon and zirconium. Crowns are made of alloys of gold, silver and palladium, with sometimes traces of nickel. Temporary crowns, fitted whilst the real ones are being made by the technician, can be made of aluminium. Metal dentures can have their bases constructed of stainless steel, which is an alloy consisting mainly of iron, carbon and molybdenum, and sometimes manganese, boron and vanadium. Much more commonly metal denture plates are made from an alloy of cobalt (mostly) and chromium. Platinum is used by dental technicians when they are making porcelain crowns, due to its very high melting point, which comes in handy in their ovens, and titanium is the metal of choice for dental implants.

Dentists use various kinds of cement, to line cavities and to protect or sedate the pulp. Many of these are compounds of zinc or calcium; while root-filling cements contain barium sulphate, so that they can be visualised on dental radiographs. Many of the tooth-cutting burs used by dentists are made from a compound of the metal tungsten, due to its strength.

Lasers have a limited place in dentistry where they can be used for cutting soft tissue or removing some forms of decay. They use the transitional metal yttrium.

Of the non-metal elements, chlorine compounds are used in cleaning, for their antibacterial qualities, iodine has a place in some tinctures while, as already mentioned, fluoride compounds have anti-cariogenic properties when bonded to tooth tissue.

Okay, that's enough chemistry for anyone! A wee bit on the application of physics now. I mentioned radiographs earlier. Why do dentists take X-rays?

The mouth lends itself very well to being X-rayed. The supporting tissues, containing bone, gum and teeth, is not very thick, and so the dose of X-ray required to 'see-through' these tissues does not have to be great. An area which shows as dark on a radiograph is therefore less dense and is called a radiolucency. Conversely, a very white area is more dense and known as a radio-opacity. Dense areas allow fewer X-rays to pass through the tissues onto the film and so the film is unaffected in these parts, and appears as white. The harder the tissue the 'whiter' it appears on a radiograph. So highly mineralised tooth enamel appears very white, whereas the inner layer of the tooth, dentine, is less mineralised and appears slightly darker; bone darker still – and patchier. Decay, or caries, shows up as a darker patch and infection around the root of a tooth likewise. These changes can be very subtle but dentists can recognise them and thus radiographs become a wonderful aid to diagnosis.

Radiographs are often taken routinely to look for early decay which would be invisible otherwise - for example, down the side of a tooth, or under a filling. They are also always taken at the start of a root-treatment, in order to assist diagnosis and to measure, accurately, the length of the root. This is so that the root-filling can be placed right to the end. Barium sulphate is added to the root-filling cement as it is radio-opaque and so appears white on a radiograph, and thus the success of its placement can be assessed. If the patient attends another practice in the future the new dentist can look at routine radiographs of a tooth and with a prescient air say "I see you have had your upper-left five root-treated, Mrs Jolly." The patient then thinks the dentist is awfully clever.

Radiographs can be used for lots of other reasons, of course, but always as a diagnostic tool. Hidden roots can be found, pathological lesions in the jaws, the angle that wisdom teeth lie at, unerupted teeth, I could go on and on, but you get the picture, I'm sure. Some real gems turn up unexpectedly. I once found what looked like a round ball-bearing, which seemed to be embedded in a chap's upper jaw, though not visible to the eye. When I asked him if he knew anything about it he replied: "oh yes somebody shot me with an airgun when I was wee."

Another chap had his upper jaw peppered with white radio-opaque splashes. Again, on cross-examining him, he was able to explain the cause.

Ten years earlier he had been badly injured in a car smash. Some of his teeth, and amalgam fillings, had been shattered, and although surgeons had cleaned him up and put his face back together again there were still traces of amalgam fragments in the soft tissues around his upper jaw and his cheek.

The dental X-ray camera can be put to other uses too. I once found an owl pellet when out walking in the hills above Paisley. Owls cough up indigestible 'fur balls' known as pellets regularly. I took it back to the practice and exposed a radiograph of it. There on the small film were the images of dozens of tiny bones and skulls from the victims the owl had consumed. I thought this was fascinating, but my nurses were unimpressed, especially when I held the film up to a patient friend of mine and told him it was his lower jaw.

For the first half of my career X-ray films were actually developed and fixed in tanks, just like photographic film. We had a large plastic cuboidal box containing tanks of developer, water and fixer. These liquids had to be changed frequently to keep up the quality of the images. This used to lead to funny conversations between the nurses, such as "...the developer's needing fixed!" In the last few years the film (which is placed in the patients' mouth in a special holder) has been replaced with a digital plate which, once exposed to the X-ray beam, is read by a computer. Once, a big-busted floosie, who was well known to the staff, came in to have a radiograph taken, and after she left I asked my nurse to process the film. She brought it into the surgery a few minutes later.

"How does she look?" I asked.

"Over developed and over exposed!" Was the reply.

Radiographs will on rare occasions pick up pathological entities that were not suspected. One Friday afternoon a young lad in his early twenties popped in for his check-up, dressed in football shirt and track suit bottoms. He was off to play 'five-a-side' football after his appointment. His mouth looked fine but he admitted to a dull ache over his lower right wisdom tooth. On closer inspection I noticed a slight blood-stained discharge from the back end of the partially erupted tooth. I took a couple of radiographs of the angle of his jaw. To my astonishment the area of his mandible directly behind and under the wisdom tooth was dark and hollow (radiolucent). It looked as though he had a cyst – a rather large one. Cysts are abnormal cavities containing (usually) fluid. They are not cancerous but can spread slowly and affect other tissues. My concern here was that his jaw bone was fragile, like an empty egg – and here he was, cheerfully about to head off to play football. I reassured him that this could be put right with a bit of clever surgery at the dental hospital, but football was out!

"It's only a wee game of 'five-a-sides'."

"Robin, one elbow to your jaw and it will snap, and your mouth will be pointing out sideways for the next six weeks."

He heeded my advice, was treated by an oral surgeon promptly and his jaw fully healed.

Dentistry wouldn't be as much fun without the patients. It is truly a privilege to be allowed to treat one's fellow human beings, and the clinician should never lose sight of that. I had many lovely, engaging and charming patients whom I grew fond of. I also knew some real pains-in-the-proverbial, but we won't go there – well maybe just a wee bit. I feel a bit ashamed to admit this now, but if I was at a party, or meeting new people socially, I rarely owned up to what I did for a living. The reason was simple: there would always be someone who on hearing that I was a dentist would immediately shove their face towards mine, pull their cheek back and demand to know what I would do with their latest dental catastrophe. When I first qualified this was fun, an honour; I felt esteemed. I soon changed my mind, and from then on, if asked in these social circles, I either charged two pints of cask ale for my advice or told him (it was usually a 'him') that I was not a dentist but an insurance salesman, keen on the make. That shut him up.

Having forty people each day walk through my door allowed me to chat to people from all walks of life. This is truly inspiring, for you can learn so much from their stories and skills. Over the years I learnt that police officers are not always fearless, and from firefighters that the number of chip-pan fires declines when the price of potatoes goes up. I was informed by pharmacists that many doctors and dentists can't spell penecillin; sorry penicillin. A flight engineer told me that sometimes mid-Atlantic both pilots sometimes have a nap at the same time. Farmers reassured me that when cows crowd around you, when your right of access crosses their field, there is nothing to fear, as they just want to lick you and sit on you. Mmmm, I'll bear that in mind but will keep running. A chef scribbled down how to make the perfect bolognaise sauce, and a plumber gave me advice on how best to unblock a toilet. I would also get to hear their life stories – some tragic some funny. A train driver described what it was like when his *Sprinter 156* hit a cow – maybe it was trying to lick his train. A bus driver described how the greatest achievement in his working career was driving past the lone passenger at a bus stop, her hand held out, because he spotted from afar that she was his wife. He didn't get his tea that night, nor anything else presumably.

I, of course, would retaliate by telling patients the difference between a common tern and an arctic tern – even if they didn't want to know. They were educated on the quickest route to cycle from Milngavie to Castlemilk – even though they lived around the corner from the practice and didn't possess a bike. I divulged the best ferry route around the Western Isles, only my route was the most convoluted, involved the greatest number of ships and incurred the greatest expense in the process. And I would bore them with the same stories and jokes; and my *Rolling Stones* story. Oh I haven't told you about that yet, have I?

Older patients could be great fun, I often found, and interestingly the older, and in fact the younger, they were the more likely they were to tell you their age. So I would frequently receive an introduction that would go something like this: "Hallo again, Mr Craig. I'm here for a check-up. I've got a bit of pain top left, but I'm 87 now, you know!" Or it could go like: "Hi mister, I'm three!"

The older patients were usually the ones who had the best stories. Many of the older people around at the time I started in practice had been through the social turmoil of the Second World War and so stories about life during the war, or when abroad during military service abounded. I found all this fascinating and often spent a good part of clinical time chatting when I should have been fixing their teeth. I met a former commando who told me he was dropped behind enemy lines and then "...shot lots of the enemy." His descriptions were a bit more graphic than these pages would allow. He was a tough character and I was particularly gentle with him.

One particular old gentleman, with an Italian name, came to me in the early 80s, for new dentures. We hit it off well and he was a very interesting gentleman. I blotted my copy book however when he started telling me that he had lost his natural teeth during the war.

"Oh dear," I said sympathetically, "and were you in the army or navy or air force?"

He leant forward and touched my arm.

"I was on the *other* side."

When working in Glasgow some years later I had several visits from a retired radiographer, who was by now *getting on* in years. But he told me a tale I have never forgotten.

He had been based in the Middle East during WW2, and working as a radiographer for the RAF. One day, a senior officer approached him and asked if he could take some of his used photographic plates away with him. These were glass plates that were coated in silver nitrate, for the purpose of recording X-rays, and which could be washed clean and re-used. My patient let him have a few dozen which were past their best, but asked what he wanted them for. The reply surprised him, wooden fake planes were being built some distance away on an airfield to fool the enemy. To render them more realistic, the glass plates were installed as 'cockpit windshields' to reflect the light and fool the enemy even more.

Some months later my patient met the senior again, and asked how the illusion had fared.

"Oh not too well, I'm afraid, one day the Luftwaffe flew over and dropped wooden, dummy bombs on them!"

A common subject that older patients liked to chat about was their experiences of dentistry when they were very young.

"It was tough going to the dentist a hundred years ago son."

"That long ago, Mr Young?"

"Yes, I'm 87 now, you know, and I was born on the kitchen table too."

Due to their memory of the aforementioned 'Good Old Days' older patients are usually quite relaxed in the chair. With their experience of life and their enthusiasm for repeating the amusing things that had happened to them over a lifetime they were usually up for a chat and a laugh whenever they appeared for their six-month check-up. The problem however was that they usually repeated the same story every time they came in (my wife says I am now suffering from this same affliction). It has to be said that men are more afflicted with this than women. So I would get to hear old Charlie's Desert Rats story, about how he lost that front tooth every time.

It seemed strange to me, but quite often a patient whom I had been treating for many years would admit at reception that they didn't know their dentist's name. They would turn up for their check-up appointment and when asked which of the two dentists in the practice they were seeing would pause.

"Eh, it's the skinny one (that would be me), the black haired one (my colleague), the younger one (either of us – we're almost exactly the same age), the good looking one (well that must be me again)."

Other more brazen patients would turn up for their first ever appointment and say:

"I'm here to see Stuart."

Mmm, are you now? I was once told, by a retired dentist, to be suspicious of patients who call you by the first name when they haven't yet had the opportunity of sitting in your chair. His warning was not without justification, I later discovered – but we won't dwell on that, except that after a prolonged course of treatment, and lots of "Hi Stuart's" my example disappeared without trace, and without paying his not inconsiderable bill. However, once patients got to know me I was very happy to be addressed by my forename, in fact, with older patients, there was something quite cute about that - it was as if they now trusted you completely.

Medical questionnaires used to elevate a few eyebrows. It is fundamentally important that the dentist knows the state of health of his/her patient. There is no point in finding out half way through an extraction that your patient suffers from haemophilia. As previously mentioned, the dentists' education in all matters medical puts them in a place where they can understand the ailments a patient may be suffering from or the nature of the medication they are taking. To provide confidential medical information from the patient a 'medical history form' is given to the patient at the start of each course of dental treatment – usually at the check-up appointment. One of the questions, usually hidden well down the list, concerned the number of units of alcohol imbibed per week. The relevance of this may, or may not, be pertinent to every course of treatment, but it was recommended that it should be included. The answers given by the patients led, I believe, to nothing short of lies, damned lies and statistics, but without the statistics bit. Chaps whom I knew practically lived in the pub would write 'three units'. Mr Dewar, when he attended to get both his teeth checked, and always exuded a piquant aroma of stale *White and Mackays* would scribble 'just the four'. One chap was commendably honest, however. He wrote 25 units. On checking over all of his answers I commented "....and 25 units per week."

He perked up in the chair, "per week? I thought you wanted per day!"

Clearly, completed medical history forms are strictly private. But it was amazing how many patients left them lying on their waiting-room seat when they were called into the surgery, even after being told to 'hand it to the dentist!' Once, when my nurse was sent out to the waiting room to retrieve such a form, she found an elderly lady reading it intently. She thought it was a new style of reading material.

"This is very interesting – I know a good cream for that, you know. Oh, and I suffer from that too, it can be very embarrassing."

Not infrequently a patient would tick every single box, thus stating they were suffering from everything on the list, from chronic heart disease to acute pregnancy. Even guys admitted to this last condition. One such over enthusiastic patient was a local GP.

"I see you have lots of diseases Dr Watson, and you're pregnant as well."

One question which used to appear on medical history forms was 'have you ever had St Vitus' Dance?' This relates to a rare condition which causes involuntary movements following a nasty bacterial infection, and has a loose connection with rheumatic conditions that are relevant to invasive dental treatment, which is why it appeared on medical forms. I never met anyone who had suffered from it, but there was a near scare once when I worked in Lanarkshire. An older lady handed over her questionnaire to me. Under the question 'have you ever had St Vitus' Dance?' she had written: "no, but I go line-dancing every Thursday night."

Patients, being mostly normal human beings, could sometimes say something which would take you completely by surprise. I always had the radio on in my surgery, to give the patient, and dentist, some background sounds to listen to. On one occasion I had a very smart-looking seventy-five year old lady in the chair when onto the radio came an item about Dolly the sheep, which had just given birth to the first mammalian clone. Between visits to her mouth she suddenly asked me, out of the blue, "did Dolly just have sex with a ram as normal?" I believe my mouth dropped open in astonishment, even wider than hers. I really had no answer to that and could only mumble that I wasn't sure but would try to find out.

On another memorable occasion a very prim lady touched my arm as I prepared to extract a tooth from her and enquired politely "Tell me, do you shake it out slowly or just wank it out?" I managed to keep a stiff upper lip, until my eye caught my dental nurse doubled up in mirth out of sight of the patient.

There were many patients whose cheery chat brightened my day. Some less so. One gentleman knew a dentist from Northumberland whom he assumed I must know. Each visit we would have the same introductory conversation.

".....I was talking to Mr Filler the other day, do you know him?"

"Eh, no. I don't know any dentists in Northumberland."

"Well he was asking for you......"

I would then listen for several minutes to stories related to the life of Mr Filler."

When my patient attended the following week for treatment we would start again.

"Mr Filler was on the phone the other day. You know him, don't you?"

"No I don't know any dentists in Northumberland."

More chat with the same details as last week followed. This would continue at every appointment, so much so that I used to prime my nurse that I was going to be informed about the mysterious Mr Filler at his every visit. And then one day I pre-empted the conversation by trumping my patient. As soon as he sat in the chair I asked. "How is Mr Filler?" This took my patient by surprise.

"Oh, eh, fine. I thought you didn't know him!"

Once the business of the check-up was over many used to feel that this was the time to stand and chat; stand, for they had now been escorted from the chair. One chap would stand and blether for half an hour if we let him. I often wondered if he would just carry on even if we all left the room. Perhaps he was lonely, and we did let him indulge for a while, but time is money in dentistry and we eventually had to nudge him towards the door. Mrs Bridges was the worst. When she was in full swing all the nurses could do to get her out the door was invent an emergency phone call from a fictitious patient which required my immediate and urgent attention. I once bumped into her in *ASDA* and just couldn't force myself away without appearing rude. Twenty minutes passed, I feigned interest, conjuring up an idea that I could collapse and pretend I'd just had a stroke. Eventually I just interrupted her and walked away, making a mental note to shop in a different supermarket.

There were a couple of individuals who wouldn't shut up during treatment. They would start a story just as the drill was poised and the only way to proceed with treatment was to shove a handful of cotton wool rolls into their mouth. After a hiatus of twenty minutes of me working they would take up the story where they had left of.

Many older patients were gems, however, and showed great respect to my time and effort and to the assistance given by the nurses. One poor old soul who had just been fitted with her new full dentures and had been given her old ones back in a bag to take away shoved them back in my hand "can these not go to charity? How about Kosova?" All I could think of to say was that Kosova had a wonderful, well-funded dental service of its own. Perhaps it does.

I recall another old dear who wandered into reception at our Glasgow practice one morning. She shuffled up and said rather loudly, as if appearing in a *Specsavers* advert "I want to make an appointment, I need new glasses."

Our receptionist kept a very straight face. "You certainly do, this is the dentist!"

We had a lovely old chap who attended every six months. He was well into his 90s and always so appreciative of anything we did for him – which wasn't much, for although he still had most of his own teeth they were in such good shape that they rarely needed any mucking about from me. Any suggestion or opinion from me was greeted with his stock phrase "First class." I could have said anything to him, and it would have received the same two-worded response.

"Your mouth looks fine, Mr S."

"First class."

"I need to do a wee filling."

"First class."

"I'm just going to take all your teeth out and put them back in upside down."

"First class."

He passed away close to his 99th birthday, and I have to admit that when his niece came to break the news to us I had a lump in my throat.

I had one cantankerous 97 year old that I made new dentures for not long before I retired. She saved most of her cantankerous rituals for her carer, who really had a hard time. At each visit she would moan about her previous dentures to the point where her carer thought it necessary to intervene and remind her that I never made her previous set and was therefore not to blame. But she would moan away, until I was up close to her, face to face, when her eyes would then give away her concealed mirth with a wink and a twinkle. Once I zoomed back, her complaints started again. On one of her visits I made a bit of a fumble trying to remove her lower denture. She pulled back and glared at me "what's the matter? They're no gonnae bite ye."

On the subject of 'face-to-face' it is clear that the practice of dentistry is a fairly intimate business. Generally, the dentist works behind the patient, from a seated position. But occasionally it is easier to stand in front and face the patient. This is particularly true when extracting a tooth from the upper jaw or from the patient's lower left jaw, or when trying in a denture, like the situation above. It is then that eye to eye contact can be, well, cosy. Usually the dentist is concentrating on what he or she is doing, and usually the patient fixes their gaze away to the side. Just occasionally, however, a patient would stare right at you, anchoring their gaze. I always found this spooky, and although focussing on the narrow gap between their lips it was clear that my every move was being studied. I could blush quite easily, and often had to withdraw to a safe distance. Back again – and the same stare. I could never figure why a patient would do that, and sometimes, when standing in front of them, face to face, I would feel an urge to giggle. Suppressing a giggle would only lead to further blushing, inevitably. I can recall times, in such situations, when I couldn't help but smile, and then the patient started smiling, and then everyone in the room was laughing. The problem was that when the same patient attended the following week both of us remembered that we had burst out laughing the last time, and that started us off again. To avoid all this, and to supress the totally unprofessional urge to giggle I would think of something sad. Little would the patient know that while apparently concentrating on the try-in of a denture their dentist was running over the Scottish football team's latest Hampden debacle or the Battle of Stalingrad in his mind.

Just as in life generally, however, you can't please everyone all of the time. I remember one bellicose lady whom I just couldn't please. I could tell as soon as she walked in for her first appointment that she was never going to be happy. For a start she had a gurn which made her look like Les Dawson, and I could see that the new dentures I was about to make for her were not going to improve that.

The dentures were made, and as soon as they were fitted I handed her the mirror for that first look (second or third look actually, for the patient gets to see the teeth before they are completed). She gave the most cursory of glances at them, paid her NHS fees and walked out without a word of thanks. Over the next three weeks she was back for adjustments, bringing a different friend with her on each occasion. I was getting nowhere. Eventually she stormed in one day and dumped a tissue containing her new dentures onto the reception counter.

"What do you really want, Mrs Dawson?"

"My money back."

"A cheque will be in the post at the end of the day." Which it truly was. My nurse was astonished.

"Why did you do that? She's a pain in the neck but you've spent all that time and money making them."

"Because, I will never have to look at her face again."

Situations like that are very undesirable but rare.

Children frequently come out with absolute gems, as we all know. As I said they often like to tell you their age too. One wee lad came in with his mum:

"Have you got toothache, Gary?"

"Yes, and I'm only five."

But sometimes it is what children are *not* saying that is funny. When doing check-ups for a family I tended to call young children into the surgery individually – I thought it was good for their confidence and helped develop a one-to-one rapport with young patients. On one occasion I seemed to have changed from my usual set-up and had two wee brothers in the surgery together; they were about six and seven. As I examined and chatted to the younger one his brother stood right beside the chair and whispered reassuring comments to his wee brother. To my surprise the lad in the chair started wriggling restlessly. I knew I wasn't hurting him, so I carried on, using my mirror to check his upper teeth. The wriggling continued. It was only when I stopped that I realised his older brother was grasping my patient's testicles tightly in his hand.

I wish I could remember all the different expressions, encouragements and thinly disguised bribes I used to get very young uncooperative patients into the chair for their check-up. Often it was clear that wee Jimmy was just not going to sit in it, and that really had to be respected. Little Chardonnay was a precocious but charming four year old whom I could tell from her stance and demeanour was not for playing ball. I tried to gently coax her to sit in the nice big comfortable chair, resorting to my full armoury of euphemisms. She stamped her foot and stood her ground.

"Look at my lovely big chair, Chardonnay, it just wants you to sit on it."

"Naw it disn'ae."

"It's a lovely, comfortable big chair."

"Naw it isn'ae."

"I'm just going to tickle your teeth."

She stood there and shook her head, and then clearly uttered "Naw yer 'no, I'll tickle them ma'sel"

Another little bright spark was in one afternoon – a wee lad of about nine, whom I had been treating since he was even smaller than nine. He surprised me on this occasion by asking why I chose to be a dentist. This was quite a profound question for one so young, and I didn't know quite how to answer, so I replied "Oh that's a long story."

He immediately returned "well just tell me half of it, then."

Children who are brought to the dentist regularly soon become great patients. One of the highlights of the job was watching a perky five year old rush into the surgery, jump up on the chair and open their mouth. When that mouth contained twenty pearly whites, all in perfect condition, it made life so much easier for everyone. One girl of about ten came in with her dad one afternoon. She was keen and threw herself onto the chair. Dad stood there, looking a bit embarrassed.

"She has a wobbly tooth, Mr Craig. I told her that it would just fall out and that she was wasting your time."

"Not at all, I am happy to see her."

He continued "...so I thought perhaps she was right and she should get a second opinion."

At this his daughter piped up "it's not a *second* opinion I want, Dad, you're not a dentist, I want a *first* opinion." I suppose she was quite right.

One young teenager climbed awkwardly into the chair one afternoon. He had noticeably grown much taller since his last appointment – which wasn't just the previous week, you understand. I felt I had to comment, "my, you've grown long legs, Declan."

"Yes", he replied, "they run in the family."

I have no idea if he meant the pun or not.

Sometimes the humour was a touch darker. I remember one chap, whose extended family were regular visitors to the practice, phoned in one afternoon. The conversation went like this:

Patient: "Hallo, I'm phoning on behalf of my dad."

Receptionist: "Okay."

Patient: "Can you tell me when his appointment is?"

Receptionist: "It's at 3.30 tomorrow."

Patient: "Well he won't make it."

Receptionist: "That's fine, does he want to re-appoint?"

Patient: "I don't think so - he died yesterday."

One hot summer's day I was drilling happily at a chap's front incisors when a tiny fly appeared from nowhere and disappeared into his mouth. My nurse and I exchanged anxious glances at each other, but the patient was oblivious. With much manipulation with her aspirator (the tube that the nurse uses to 'sook' away water and debris) the offending beastie was expunged - at least we think it was. Unbelievably this happened again some time later; it must have been a hot summer. This time the fly made its entrance while I was taking a radiograph of a young woman. Again she didn't notice, but this time I couldn't find it. When the film was developed there was the little rascal's image next to her upper molar. OK, I just made that last bit up.

As you will discover later on, we occasionally took our staff on day trips – to boost their morale! One March we took them to the Ayr Races. There, at the track side, I spotted a bookmaker that I knew - in fact I had taken three teeth out of him just a few days earlier. He spotted me and immediately engaged in that desultory and seemingly arbitrary gesticulation of tic-tac. I wondered if he was communicating with me, and a glance around me confirmed that he was indeed. I nodded back to him - and he persisted. Was he was giving me the odds against the favourite in the next race? Not having the slightest clue about tic-tac I just grinned inanely back at him. He raised his arm, pointed to his cheek, raised three fingers with the other hand, appeared to give a thumbs-up, and on it went. Eventually I went over to him and told him that I was sorry but I didn't understand bookmakers' speak. Now he laughed.

"No, what I'm trying to tell you is that following the three teeth you took out last week my gum now feels fine and all is well."

I certainly got the wrong end of the stick there, but sometimes the patient did. A female patient of mine had just run the Glasgow Marathon. She seemed understandably pleased with herself for having trained thoroughly and then completing the course. I was well impressed and wondered how long she had taken to run it, so I asked:

"What did you do it in?"

She looked quizzically at me and replied "Eh, T-shirt and shorts."

We can all get our words muddled up. A lady once came in for her check-up and told me that she had had "...an attack of sensibility." I think she meant sensitivity, so that's what I treated her for. A different young woman appeared at our reception one morning and told the receptionist she "had an appointment for a ketchup!"

On more than one occasion a patient came in and announced that they "....had a hole in their bottom." It was at times like these that I gave the patient a lecture on why we refer to upper and lower teeth – not top and bottom.

There were times when I didn't correctly pick up what a patient was saying. Mr Tote came in with toothache one Monday morning. I could tell he was nervous, and with the mouth he had he had good reason. I asked him where he worked, and thought he replied 'a pet shop'. So off I went on a pre-treatment prattle about the succession of budgies we used to have as pets when I was a lad. He listened bemused as I gave our family history of pets, updating him to the guinea pigs and the rabbits we currently had in domestic captivity. Only when I asked him if he could bring in a couple of goldfish at his next appointment did he stop me.

"I work in a BET shop!"

"Oh, any tips for the Grand National?"

Patients often turned up bearing gifts, not necessarily goldfish. Perhaps it was bribery, but I always gave them the benefit of the doubt. Mostly they were for the nurses, but just once in a while I would be on the receiving end. Biscuits, chocolates and cake would walk in the door. One lady brought me a home-baked Victoria sponge at every visit. I used to insist she got a check-up once a fortnight! Obviously, being a dental practice, we had to biologically dispose of it all – just how I cannot reveal, but it was definitely biological! I mean, we could hardly eat it, could we?

Around 1990 I did a small filling for a Chinese lady. I never treated her again, and yet each year, just before Christmas, she brought in a veritable sack of Oriental goodies. Waving cats, pandas, biscuits, glass turtles, paper fans, bits of the Great Wall and so on, I could have opened my own shop. I accepted it all, and took it as a good omen.

I received Christmas cards from Muslim patients, Easter cards from Jewish patients and postcards from patients who had had to seek treatment while on holiday in Spain. One Asian lady came in with a tub of pakora. It was so delicious we practically ate it in front of her. She seemed delighted and so regularly showed up with samples of homemade curry and nan bread – so frequently, in fact, that we practically gave her orders whenever she was due in for treatment.

"We're just phoning to let you know your check-up is due next week Mrs Singh, oh, and we'll have two portions of Rogan Josh, some fish pakora and a couple of chapatis, please."

One chap worked for a well- known Uddingston biscuit maker, and one day appeared with a carton of their goodies – merely because at his last visit I had commented on how much I liked them but hadn't eaten one for weeks! His treatment was particularly painless that day. The girls' eyes lit up with delight, evidently thinking that there were several fulfilling tea-breaks ahead of them. I sympathised, but ultimately did the right thing, for the sake of their teeth. I took the box home and ate the whole lot myself. I saw it as an act of self sacrifice.

When I retired I was overwhelmed by the bottles of malt I received – overcome almost! It has taken me a long time to get through them, in fact may I just pause here to refill my glass.... all very kind and much appreciated.

When I first qualified gloves were not worn by dentists, nor their nurses. That seems odd now, looking back. Throughout my time as a student, and for the first couple of years in dental practice, gloves did not exist; I can still remember the sticky feeling of blood on my hands. Obviously we all washed our hands thoroughly between procedures, but it wasn't until the AIDS scare of the mid 80s that operating gloves became *de rigeur*, and the first batches I tried were poor quality. One day one of my regular patients turned up at my first Glasgow practice with several large boxes. He had come across dozens of gloves, possibly off the back of a lorry, and wanted to enter into some kind of financial deal for them. I had a look at a sample. They were the kind that would come in handy for washing the dishes or pruning the roses, so I had to decline – much to my patient's disappointment.

Gloves soon improved dramatically in quality and very soon it became unthinkable to touch anyone's mouth without wearing a pair. An increase in allergies from latex-based materials led to non-allergenic nitrile gloves becoming widely used in dentistry. These are usually bright blue, but I went through a spell wearing black ones, whom one lady patient of mine termed my 'doctor death gloves'. I still have a box, which I now use for frightening the grandchildren.

I mentioned the comedy film *Little Shop of Horrors* several pages back, in relation to extraction instruments. The fascination that actor Bill Murray portrayed so enthusiastically in the film could actually be based on fact. Yes, I treated a patient who was similarly, if not quite so effusively beguiled, by my array of 'tools'. He was a guy, of course; only males get absorbed by technicalities such as the purpose of each implement in the toolkit. On his first visit Mr Jewson sat boldly upright when my nurse laid the standard tray of instruments on my little operating table.

"My, what are all these for? Please tell."

"Well, this is a mouth mirror, then there's a probe, tweezers, flat plastics - actually made of steel, but used to smooth filling materials when still in their pliable medium - a couple of excavators..."

"Stop right there, excavators?"

"Eh, yes, they are used to remove soft decay."

"Carry on."

"This is an amalgam plugger, and this a burnisher."

"Goodness, but you must have lots more in those drawers there?"

I'm getting a bit suspicious now, but played along, and showed him the back-up kit – full of hoes, chisels, Jacquettes, sickle scalers....Mr Jewson's eyes lit up, like a five year old on Christmas Day.

I stopped short of pulling out all the surgical instruments, but he had evidently seen plenty. During future visits to the practice he would then demand to know the technicalities of each procedure.

"Are you going to use the enamel chisel today on my upper-left seven, there's deep cervical caries there that needs excavating? Then I think a glass-ionomer filling would suffice. Some lignocaine first, I presume?"

Mr Jewson had been studying his dental book, it would seem. The temptation to hand him a hand mirror and suggest he took a leaf from Mr Bean's book and fill his tooth himself was almost overpowering. Once I had restored his tooth, *my way*, I looked at my notes to find out what this endearing chap did for a living. He was a firefighter. So at his next appointment I was well armed.

"Big fire last night, Mr J, I take it you were there. Did you have to use the Scania 1000 gallon tanker with the 13.5 metre ladder? And was the 87 mm hose sufficient or did you have to utilise the HVP (that's 'high volume pump', by the way?"

While he stared incredulously at me I quickly added "...or did you just call *Thunderbirds*?

NURSES SAY THE FUNNIEST THINGS

Over the years it has been a privilege to work with a group of people who were almost invariably very nice folk – dental nurses; usually, but not exclusively, young women. The vast majority were great fun to work with and very caring to their patients. Clearly no dentist could work without the support of a good dental nurse. Many were very loyal and stayed with us for years – and are still friends with us and with each other.

Nurses are in prime position to know and understand the way their dentist works, as they sit alongside him or her for hour after hour every day. Like most practitioners I am a creature of habit and would come out with the same stock expressions and quips, hour by hour. The girls who had the pleasure of my company over all these years must have cringed when they knew one of my standard utterances was coming up. For example, in a woeful attempt to relax a patient whom I was about to suture (sew) up following a minor surgical procedure I would always say, once started: "just as well I was at my embroidery class last night!" On one such occasion, I had popped out of the surgery to fetch a 'sewing kit' and my nurse had suitably primed the patient. As I leant over to start the suturing both nurse and patient, in unison, blurted out: "just as well you were at your embroidery class last night!"

I tried to use appropriate humour in the surgery - a few laughs can make the day trundle along with less friction and more jollity. If that can involve the patient too then all the better. There were many times, however, I feel ashamed to admit, when the patient was not included in the joke.

In the late 80s we had a lady who was a very regular visitor, in fact she often attended several times – a week! She was overweight, and rather slow moving, and also rather slow at understanding any advice or instruction given to her. She also suffered from trismus - an inability to open her mouth very wide. Oh, and her teeth weren't great either, but we were trying to sort that out. In short, she was a difficult lady to deal with for several reasons, but I was patient (it wasn't easy) and I tried my best. There was a spell when she was literally at our door every other day – not necessarily in pain, but with some new problem or another. One morning she came shuffling into the surgery and gradually swung her bulk onto my chair. I was working with one of our bubbliest nurses Tammy that morning, who always had a smile and a chuckle. She was standing behind the dental chair, out of sight of the patient, waiting to assist.

"What can I do for you this morning Mrs Doddle?" Trying to make my voice sound as enthusiastic as possible.

"Before you start, Mr Craig, I want to tell you that this will be my last visit here, I am moving to England."

Behind the chair Tammy gave her best impression of the Riddler from *Batman* with the biggest grin she could muster and started jumping up and down with joy. Much as I tried to bite my lip, as Mrs D started on today's menu of symptoms, I started to smile. I held it together for a few seconds, but Tammy's animations were hitting home. My grin only widened; Mrs Doddle paused.

"Have I said something funny, Mr Craig?"

This only made Tammy more animated. Pursing my lips together, and feeling my face turn bright red, I could only stammer out "oh no, not at all." Tammy got sent to make the tea and I dealt with Mrs D – for the last time!

It will shock and appal the reader to discover here that sugary snacks were occasionally consumed at the practice; not frequently – just about every hour or so, that's all. It's shocking I know, but one cannot constantly practise what one preaches. Energy levels would drop, and a wee snack would help get the cup of tea down. Some of our nurses, over the years, could be very indulgent and wee Geraldine was particularly guilty. In the days before computerised appointment books we had a huge, broad ledger at reception into which appointments were written in pencil. One day Geraldine was at reception and happily munching her way through a bag of *Maltesers*. A patient appeared suddenly out of my colleague's surgery and presented unexpectedly at the reception desk. Geraldine jumped, and slammed the book shut, hiding her bag of goodies.

"I've to make another appointment, please, Geraldine."

"Oh really, would you like to phone in?"

"Eh, well I'm here, so I could just make it just now."

"Oh, okay then."

As Geraldine raised the ledger up and opened it at the correct page a dozen *Maltesers* rolled out from the bottom onto the desk, to the astonishment of the patient.

Still on a confectionary note, a patient drew my attention to what he thought was a hilarious incident that happened just outside the front door of the practice. The door was locked, as it was lunchtime, but my patient arrived ten minutes early for his appointment and tried the door handle. Just at that moment, our dental nurse Brenda opened the door from the inside, obviously heading out.

"Oh, hallo Mr Promptly, you're a wee bit early. But I'll let you inside in five minutes, I'm just popping out for some sweeties for the girls!"

Mr Promptly thought this was so funny he passed it on to me – and I passed it on to Brenda.

"You need to be careful, Brenda, this doesn't show a good example. 'Nipping out for sweeties!'

"I'm sorry, Stuart, that was silly of me."

"I mean, what must the patient have thought?"

"I'm sorry. It won't happen again. Here, have half a macaroon bar."

"Oh, okay."

Inevitably the love-life of the current group of dental nurses at the practice would be aired around the staff room. At times this could be entertaining; sometimes astonishing. My colleague and I would sometimes be asked for advice, as if we were some kind of relationship therapists. Our nurse, Patricia, had a particularly colourful love-life (so the other nurses told us) and had been accused a few times, by her colleagues, of 'jumping in with both feet.' I never knew if that was an in-joke or a euphemism, but one particular morning she came to work looking rather glum. I sat with her a while as she drank a cup of tea and swallowed a packet of *Revels*. It turned out that her boyfriend of two months had just 'chucked' her. I tried to offer advice.

"Have you been guilty of doing something with both feet?" I enquired, trying to be whimsical.

She thought for a moment, then replied in the affirmative.

"What was it?" I prompted.

"Jumping in head first."

There was more than one occasion when a male patient had seemingly fallen in love, instantly, with one of our nurses. One was Sammy, whose eyes followed Natalie around the surgery absorbing her every move. Natalie pretended not to notice – but a dentist notices every little thing. When she leaned over him to start aspirating I had to quickly throw a long bib over him.

During the early days at the Glasgow practice, at each of his visits, Mr Keen would always ask if Susie would be helping me that day. Susie would charm him, oblivious to his developing motive. One day he asked me if Susie had a boyfriend. I pointed out that she did, but added that she was 20 years old, while he was approaching 67! We never saw him again.

Dental nurses love when moments of light humour punctuate the working day –sometimes they go out their way to create their own moments. We once had a nurse, whom we shall call Jennifer, who was often boasting to her colleagues on the quality, and shall we say animation, of her sex life. These were conversations which I can assure you I and my colleague took no part in. One week in particular, Jennifer could be heard regaling stories about her newly acquired handcuffs. Her colleagues around her, who showed an interest, were instructed on how these could be applied, and in what circumstances. I closed my ears, of course. A week later she appeared at work with two bruised stripes across the inner side of each wrist. I said nothing. In mid-morning she was working in my surgery when a policeman patient of mine arrived for his appointment, in uniform, and sat on the chair for whatever procedure I had planned. Jennifer chatted brightly to him for a moment or two, and then, to my horror asked to see his handcuffs. He smiled, and produced them.

"I've got handcuffs too, you know," said Jennifer.

"Oh no, Jennifer, not here," I thought.

She then showed him her wrists.

"I'll tell you how I got these," she proclaimed.

I had to speak up. "Oh no Jennifer, not here!"

She looked at me curiously, and continued. "I was taking a chicken out of the hot oven last night and the grill briefly touched my arms – look I've got two sets of burns."

Even the bobby in the chair looked relieved.

Geraldine was a great nurse and working with her was a pleasure, most of the time. When working in the surgery, however, she did have a habit of dropping instruments and materials. Her movements about the practice were punctuated with the unmistakable sound of breaking glass. She would frequently mix a measure of alginate impression material and hold her spatula out for me, only for us to watch as the new mix blobbed onto the floor.

"I see we're taking an impression of the lino again, Geraldine."

Filling materials, paper cups, polishing brushes, extraction forceps and amalgam would all meet a similar fate. I once suggested to her that we should put all the instruments and materials onto the floor to begin with.

Her turn of phrase was often a joy. She could be heard telling patients on the phone during a frenetic morning that she was "....fitting the patients in at all angles." I could just imagine folk walking in crouched double or bending over backwards.

Her *piece de resistance* was one apparently quiet Monday morning when a patient asked why we appeared not to be busy.

"Oh we will be," replied Geraldine, "this is just the storm before the tea cup."

She always kept us entertained. On looking at the newspaper one lunchtime she pointed at the headline about an impending famine in Niger.

"That's shocking," she declared, "that's obscene, they shouldn't print words like that, it's banned!" I had to point out that Niger was a country in West Africa. A few pages further on she was appalled to read that the council were intending to run a new road very close to where she lived.

"I'm not happy with that – I'm going to sign a partition."

Inevitably there would be moments when relationships were strained. Sometimes the working session was just too busy and stresses could build up. On one such occasion, on a mild September morning, I was having a stressful time. Our receptionist Wendy was typing furiously at the office computer and as usual, despite it being 25C in the practice, the fan heater was on full blast. It is a curious thing that dental nurses always feel the cold. I had turned it down a few times that particular morning but strangely it always seemed to turn itself back up again. Taking my frustration about something in the surgery out to the office, I went over to Wendy's desk and asked when those reports she had been working on all morning would be ready. Noticing the heater blasting out once again I reached down and felt for the plug in the wall.

"And another thing...it is far too hot in here!" With that I yanked the plug out of the wall, only to watch in dismay as the heater stayed on and Wendy's computer screen went blank.

She looked at me coolly and muttered "that was a whole morning's work."

We didn't laugh about it then but we can now.

Geraldine soon came up with another gem one day, after a firm had written to us asking if we wanted to pay them for recycling empty or part used local anaesthetic cartridges. She thought this was a good idea "....it'll save the environment, help Greenpeace and will mean they can be refilled and recycled instead of putting them down manholes."

Playing tricks on each other could be such fun. When Geraldine had only been working with us a couple of months our head nurse Tammy approached me with a naughty idea for a bit of fun. Geraldine was keen on drawing and had asked Tammy if she could borrow, for one night, the big electric pencil sharpener we had in reception (remember, in those days appointments were written into our book in pencil, so a sharp pencil was essential for the running of the practice). Near closing-up time Tammy told her to put it in her bag, and then approached me. So just before six o'clock closing, when our girls were donning their coats, I asked all our staff to gather round for an important chat.

"Ladies, I met a colleague the other day who told me a sorry tale of one of his staff stealing from the practice. Now I know we can trust you all here, but we feel that it might be good practice to have an occasional bag search, of everyone, so that we all feel we are being treated fairly. So tonight's the night, if you don't mind lining up."

At that poor Geraldine turned the same colour as her orange hair and stuttered: "well I'll tell you right now, I've got the pencil sharpener in my bag." She looked mortified. "Tammy said I could take it."

"No I didn't," said Tammy, and then the joke was out. How cruel.

The names of all the patients attending on each day were written out in a chronological list for the dentist, so that he could see who was coming in that day, at what time and for what reason. This is known as the Day List. One April Fools' Day I got the girls to compile a spurious Day List for my colleague. We wrote out a list of his least favourite patients, requiring the most awkward treatments, and in the shortest possible appointment times. When he came in, he glanced at it without comment, and settled down for a challenging day – such was his professionalism. I would have run back out the door. He waited a year and got his own back, however. Exactly twelve months later I was totally panicked when the receptionist told me the chief of Greater Glasgow Health Board was on the phone wanting to speak to me urgently about the aforementioned Mrs D. I donned my usual hue of flustered pink and headed to the phone, only to be greeted by much cackling from the extension line in the surgery next door.

We played the odd trick on the nurses, of course, why wouldn't we? They all loved going out for dinner at Christmas time – why wouldn't they? They weren't paying! Aware that Geraldine loved garlic mushrooms and lasagne (she apparently never ate anything else when she went out for dinner) I arranged with our restaurant in advance to have a special menu made up just for her. The five starters were all variations on garlic mushrooms: creamy garlic mushrooms, stuffed garlic mushrooms, garlic-free garlic mushrooms. The mains were all similarly combinations of lasagne: lasagne with peas, lasagne without peas, lasagne with mince, veggie lasagne. She was duly handed the menu as soon as she was seated while we all watched her, sucking in our cheeks to stop smiling.

"Oh good they've got garlic mushrooms and lasagne," she exclaimed. In fact the chef had specially made both dishes for her that evening. But I think she chose soup and steak pie instead.

The girls got their own back, on several occasions. I used to cycle to work – locking my bike to a post out in the yard behind the practice. One lunchtime I came out to get it and it had disappeared. I rushed back inside, shouting "someone's stolen my bike!"

Much laughter gave away their treachery: they had hidden it in the butcher's shop next door, there it was, hanging from a meat hook. On another occasion the rim of my tea mug was liberally coated in topical anaesthetic gel, rendering the tea undrinkable and giving me numb lips for half an hour.

The girls' finest moment (they would claim) was when they scared the proverbial out of me when I returned from lunch one afternoon. Many of our dental supplies arrived in large cardboard boxes – big enough to hide little Geraldine in. She was tucked away inside one, in the cramped confines of our staff room. As I quickly changed from cycling gear to my clinical togs out she popped, like an orange jack-in-the-box while I was in a state of semi-decency. I got such a fright I didn't speak to her for two days – so she now tells me, but I think she exaggerates.

We never played tricks on patients, that wouldn't have been professional, but I once saw a perfect opportunity for a prank on a patient of mine outside of the practice environment. I was just finishing up at the hairdressers when a glance in the mirror revealed a chap I regularly treated being shown into a chair further up the shop. I couldn't resist it. I walked up to behind the chair, winked at the hairdresser and took the gown from him. Placing it over my patient's shoulders I looked at him in the mirror.

"What can I do for you today, Mr Baldy?"

The poor chap looked at me in the mirror and after a couple of confused seconds shot skywards. Yes, he did remain a patient.

Geraldine was back in action again not long after this. Mrs Blair was in the chair, and Mrs Blair was very well endowed in the....eh...bosom department. On the completion of the treatment her attributes were clearly in Geraldine's mind, for as she prepared to remove the protective bib she announced "that's us finished Mrs Blair, let me take this boob from you."

As any of you who have been to a dentist will know - and I hope that's all of you – dental nurses have a crucial role to play in assisting the dentist. Apart from chatting and relaxing the patients there are instruments and materials to look out and hand to the dentist during the various procedures. When nurses are trained to a high level they can become very involved with the actual treatment – an arrangement known as 'four handed dentistry'. One of their main roles is to aspirate water, saliva or any other material away from inside the patient's mouth. This clears debris, leaves a clean field of operation and stops the patient from drowning. Powerful suction is used for this and the hand-held tube employed by the nurse is known as an *aspirator*. Patients used a variety of nouns when referring to this tube, whatever came into their head to best describe it: the 'sooker' the 'tube' the 'cleaner-ooter'. One day a middle-aged chap, on feeling his mouth filling up, turned to my nurse and asked if she could give him 'a wee suck out.' He said it quite innocently, but nurses being nurses she had to spend the rest of the session looking the other way. I aspirated!

For a good part of my career I was a keen cyclist, often heading off somewhere down the coast on my half day. Half day was a Wednesday, when many dentists traditionally play golf; I liked to cycle. One Wednesday I brought my new bicycle into the surgery to show off to the nurses, and any patients who might be lingering. I was heading for Largs, and had scrubbed the bike the night before so that it looked its best. It gleamed and sparkled, and I had adorned it with tool kit, phone-holders, pump, map holder, lock, water bottle and a triangular bag slung below the top tube, containing my lunch. I gestured to the girls to step forward and admire it, and to ask anything they wanted. They stood around, silently, looking at my machine. Eventually Cherie spoke up:

"What's in your sandwiches?"

We held weekly 'practice meetings' with our staff, for a half hour every Monday. This enabled them to air any problems and make suggestions. Likewise the dentists could shout back at them. No, seriously, it was a great way to sort problems out and make positive contributions to the running of the practice. Here we could air any gripes, come up with suggestions as to how the surgeries could run better and allow the dentists to listen to their hard-working staff. Minutes would be written down from these meetings and logged into a notebook. All the ideas forthcoming would be added, and many of them acted upon. These meetings genuinely helped smooth the waters when things went wrong or when Mary had had a fall-out with Betty. Generally most comments referred to when the nurses could get new uniforms and where we were going for our Christmas lunch. Common gripes were patients being put in the wrong dentist's appointment book and the dentists running late.

I kept the minute books and include a few gems from them here. The numbers refer to the month and year of the meeting in question and the comments in brackets are mine:

2/95 "Tammy had wind." (Whether this disrupted the meeting is not duly noted).

6/95 "Wanda wondering what to wear when she gets fat." (Wanda was four months pregnant).

1/96 "Cherie sent trousers back and is painting her legs." (I think this refers to her uniform).

2/96 "Fixer on doors turning paint blue."(The fixer, used in our developing machine, could linger on the operator's gloves if not rinsed properly, and when it came into contact with white painted doors left a pale blue smudge. This was an ongoing problem and we seriously considered just painting the whole practice cobalt blue).

1/98 "Bernadette's new uniform looks nice but keep the same legs." (I can't now remember who Bernadette was, but she seemed to have nice legs).

3/98 "Nurses to shave every day." (We had two male nurses at the time, so I think this refers to them).

5/98 "Children should always be seen and patients to be treated better" (I couldn't agree more!)

1/03 "Doorbell stolen." (Indeed it was – more than once).

1/03 "If any more woodlice found in reception let dentists know." (What we would have done about it is anyone's guess).

2/04 "Get headrest covers as smelly patients are sitting on them." (I told the patients so many times not to sit on the headrests! Especially if they were smelly).

3/04 "Ask all patients about possibility of being pregnant - not men though!" (We didn't ask nuns either).

12/04 "Discussed Sheila's injury yesterday - her acrylic nail came off on ladders. She was taken to hospital and they put a bandage on it." (The ladder was used to access the loft where we stored lots of dental goodies - and a few patients in case the appointment book became quiet).

8/04 "Bernadette stabbed with scaler." (She frequently did this, hopefully not on her nice legs this time).

10/05 "Hot water tap to get willy." (Mmmm, I think there is one word and one punctuation mark missing from this. Our plumber was called Willy and I believe the line should read "Hot water tap burst, to get Willy." Either that, or the tap needed one of those rubbery pipe attachments).

1/06 "Sheila would like to know why "its (sic) tooth whitening and not teeth whitening." (I really have no idea, I usually whitened them one at a time).

3/06 "Too much toilet paper being used by Wanda." (Well she was pregnant!)

6/06 "To be careful passing Stuart's chair when he's giving an injection." (This was after I stabbed four patients in the neck on a busy Monday as the enlarging Wanda squeezed past my chair).

11/06 "Practise Inspection, someone will be coming to cheek up" (Someone needs to cheek their spelling.)

Occasionally we took them out of the practice for a wee treat. One of these was to the dental lab we used, so that they could meet the technicians face to face and see how they went about producing all their fine work. The lab owner gave up his lunch hour to accommodate us, as he explained how to make casts from the impressions, make acrylic dentures and fabricate crowns. Once he had finished we gathered around his worktop and he invited questions from the girls.

"Ask anything at all."

Silence.

"Nothing?"

Cherie cleared her throat. "What have you got in your sandwiches?"

In the mid-noughties my colleague and I became more adventurous and organised a series of annual day-trips for our staff, aimed at keeping their morale high! The girls loved this, or at least told us they did. We took them on paddle steamer *Waverley*, we spent a day in The Trossachs and we took them to a production of the ballet *Swan Lake* at the Theatre Royal in Glasgow. Not all on the same day, of course.

In October 2006 we flew down to Stansted Airport at the unearthly hour of 0600 for a visit to a dental exhibition held in the ExCel Centre in London. After a morning spent browsing the stalls, collecting catalogues and filling our bags with free tubes of toothpaste and mouthwash we headed upstream. We took a boat trip on the Thames and then had one complete revolution of the London Eye. All good fun, until it was time to catch our Stansted Express train from Liverpool Street Station, back to the airport for our flight home. The destination board at the station had all its lights twinkling red; all trains were suspended due to a signalling failure. We were stranded. The idea of wandering from station to station looking for a train that would expedite our journey didn't appeal so we just had to sit and wait. We eventually got to Stansted – but the Ryanair bird had flown. We had to re-book alternative flights for the next day, and find a hotel for six of us. The girls really loved this *one*! My colleague and I were overjoyed too, well it was a pleasure to spend a further £600 on a day out!

Patients' names can create a problem – they shouldn't, but they do. We had a lovely wee lady who was a regular attender at our Lanarkshire practice. She was a sweet thing but unfortunately she didn't smell very sweet, for she worked at a nearby fish shop, and yes, you've guessed it, she smelled of haddock. We were well used to this, of course, and naturally we gave her the appellation Mrs Fish; but not to her face. One Tuesday morning she popped into reception unannounced, wanting a denture adjustment, but her visit coincided, regrettably, with a new girl, Jane, starting with us. Our receptionist stuck her head round the door of my surgery and said "Mrs Fish has come in, she wonders if you could adjust her denture." I nodded and Jane scribbled something on my day-list page.

Now Mrs Fish's real name was McDonald. Well for the sake of privacy it wasn't that either, but we'll just call her that. In she came and ten minutes later she stood up from the chair much relieved.

"Thank you Mr Craig, that feels a lot better."

"You're welcome," I replied.

Jane chose this moment for her flash of glory "nice to meet you, Mrs Fish."

Fortunately Mrs Fish, I mean McDonald, was as deaf as a trout, as well as piquant. Interestingly over the years I had patients by the name of Salmon, Pike and Turbot.

Other names occasionally gave us problems with pronunciation. We are all familiar with the very Scottish ones, as long as you could sort out the Finlay

Camerons from the Cameron Findlays. Asian names were quite easy, African ones sometimes problematic but the strangest were some Irish ones. I heard some unusual articulation of names which when uttered didn't seem to match with the spelling. Put that down to our ignorance. We had a Polish lady whose name our receptionist couldn't get her tongue around. Each time she attended the practice I was reminded of the Wimbledon umpire who got his knickers in a twist every time Miss Navratilova was on court. He just couldn't get her name out.

Some dentists have had wonderfully apt names. There used to be a Mr Gummers practising not far from where I lived. I've also heard of a Dr Fang, Dr Swallow and, somewhat inevitably, Mr Payne. I don't believe the authenticity of Mr D. Kay or Dr Phil McCavity however.

I am reminded of a particular 'name' problem that I heard from one of my nieces, who worked at Glasgow Airport several years ago. Mr and Mrs Knott and family were off to Palma de Mallorca, but hadn't appeared at the departure gate, as the flight was ready to close. Out went the announcement:

"Will the family Knott going to Palma please proceed urgently to gate 26."

A hundred and fifty people showed up at the gate: "we're not going to Palma!"

STRANGER THINGS HAVE HAPPENED

As I mentioned earlier I liked to have background music in the surgery. This was usually the radio – tuned into Radio 2 – but was often music from my own eclectic catalogue of cassettes. The patient only got to listen to Cold Play or Bowie at their six-monthly visits but my poor staff had to endure my favourites daily, and so they got to know every lyric. I stored a dozen or so cassettes on a shelf behind my chair in the surgery and would occasionally pop one into the mini-system I had. This led to one very spooky moment back in 2010. I had just finished a treatment for a chap I knew well from his many years as a patient. Nothing was playing on my system at the time, but we got chatting about music. The ages of surviving Beatles Paul McCartney and Ringo Starr cropped up. Just as we were musing over this a book on the shelf behind me shifted. It fell sideways and knocked one cassette off onto the floor between us with a clatter. We jumped in fright, then I bent down to pick it up. It was *Abbey Road*, by the Beatles, of course.

Flukes like that could fill an entire book, but there is one other unusual coincidence that I feel I have to share with you, despite its unsavoury nature. Treating one's fellow human beings can have its sublime moments, but there can be times when the biological entities that we are can fashion less appealing situations. On two occasions in my career I had to clean excrement off my dental chair following the visit of anally compromised patients. I won't go into the reasons why these little accidents had happened, but I felt it was my duty to attend to them myself, rather than delegate my nurse. But here is the strange thing, despite a total of 33 years in practice, amounting to at least 7500 days in the surgery, both these incidents happened on the *same* day: one in the morning and one in the afternoon! A new girl had just started that week at the practice; by the end of that day she must have wondered if she had made the right choice of career. Her face was a picture when the latter patient, rising from the chair completely unaware of the devastation he had left behind, headed for the door with a cheery "see you again next week!"

While we are on the subject, my colleague and I frequently reminded our staff that both of us were happy to attend to the little unpleasant jobs that occasionally popped up, requiring attention. I was very good at making tea, while my pal always lent himself to cleaning out the toilet after a certain patient of his – a man of the cloth, I might add – had vacated it. Clearly the poor chap had a touch of the old bladder trouble, for he always paid at least two visits during any of his appointments at the practice and always seemed to hose the toilet bowl down, in the manner of *Fireman Sam*. At least when my chum emerged with his rubber gloves after re-sanitising it there was a cup of tea waiting for him.

The girls that came to work for us as dental nurses soon developed a strong stomach for the less glamourous aspects of dentistry, with one exception. One poor girl started at 9 o' clock on a Monday morning and lasted till half past ten. Watching my colleague carry out a rather enthusiastic and effusive scaling she turned green and quietly left. She didn't just leave the surgery – she collected her coat and left the building. We phoned her sympathetically later but she declined to return the next day to try again. "I think I have made a mistake," she said.

With training and growing experience there are few situations, like that one, which the dentist, or nurse, finds disagreeable. Inevitably there were some unsavoury situations which we were confronted with. I was always puzzled when wee Alec turned up for his routine appointment and jumped up on the chair with a face covered in dried spaghetti bolognaise. If it were my child I think I would have wiped their face before bringing them to the dentist. Likewise a face-full of bogies is not particularly pleasant either. I used to hand a tissue to the mum or dad and suggest they wipe a nose. One dad failed to take the hint and used it to wipe his own nose. Most people would brush their teeth before visiting the dentist, and may I take the unusual step here of thanking all of those who did. I mean, who would go to the chiropodist without washing their feet first? Well, I suppose some would, probably the same people who wouldn't think to brush their teeth before visiting their dentist.

At one of our frequent practice meetings one of the girls suggested we get a coffee machine for the waiting room – to keep the patients awake. When I pointed out that thereafter every patients' breath would smell of stale coffee she retracted the idea.

Personal hygiene, or a lack of it, would raise its malodorous head frequently. It was essential that dentist and nurses were immaculately turned out, of course. Clean uniforms, neat hair, freshly shaved......and the same goes for the guys too! The patients were allowed to turn up in any state they desired. We got used to the 'regulars' who seemed to wash in soup instead of soap. I briefly worked as an associate in Ardrossan. The principal of the practice, Mr McPhee, was a really nice chap and one day his nurse asked if I could see one of his patients as he was busy.

"Can you see Miss Campbell?" She asked, supressing a grin – or was it a grimace.

"Of course."

"Be warned, it's been raining," she continued.

"What do you mean?"

"She always smells worse when she's wet." I soon appreciated what she meant. It was quite difficult doing a filling at arm's length.

Other odours, like cheap perfume or after shave would also make me flinch, on occasion. Tiny Mrs Rose would always exude the concentrated essence of several gardens, while Mr Stratos must have had daily baths in the blue stuff.

On the subject of my brief spell at Ardrossan, Mr McPhee, always one for relating a good tale, suggested I take a stroll down the High Street at lunchtime and look in a particular newsagent's window. Apparently a lady from the town had a starring role within the pages of a monthly soft porn magazine under the category 'Readers' Wives'. The enterprising newsagent had a copy placed in his window, with an attached note indicating: 'of local interest.' I never found out if she was a patient at the practice, or not.

Sadly, other emanations often hinted at a decline in a patient's overall well-being. Seeing a smart, well turned out, regular client gradually exhibit such a declivity was a poignant reminder that we are all vulnerable. It was always an honour to help such people; perhaps even just smoothing a rough tooth or patching a cavity in a molar that was evidently beyond repair – just like the patient.

Working in close proximity to patients' hair could be interesting. I found suspicious freckles I suggested got checked out. I sometimes could tell the make of shampoo being used and I watched little worming lice creep across, trying to find a new host. One lady, with striking, long, jet black hair asked me not to be put back in the chair in case her wig fell off. I wouldn't have known it was a wig, in fact, having treated many patients undergoing chemotherapy it was remarkable how difficult it was to tell if that was a wig or real hair on their head.

Hair in other places can be most interesting. Bristle-nosed ageing men, for example. One chap looked as though he had a dead badger up each nostril – I don't know how he manged to breathe. I even noticed hair on the side of a chap's tongue once. This was developing on a small skin graft, used to repair a defect following surgery for an oral cancer.

At our Glasgow practice I wanted to have a large photograph for the ceiling that patients reclined in the chair could look at as they sat there, nice and relaxed. When a friend of mine gave me a poster-sized photograph of paddle steamer *Waverley*, that he took while hanging off the Erskine Bridge, I knew I had the ideal image. So I pinned it to the ceiling. This produced much comment over the years, as occupants in the chair looked up at the ship, when the photograph suggested they should be looking down at it. I then considered having a poster made of me looking down at a patient, mirror and probe in hands, taken from the patients' perspective. This meant that while examining them they would see a double image of me poised over them. Nobody in the practice thought this was a good idea.

"It's bad enough them looking at your face hovering over them without seeing the same image on the ceiling," my nurse kindly pointed out. I wouldn't have minded her comments, but she had only been in the job three days.

There was a blank wall facing my dental chair which I decided to adorn with shelves full of silly memorabilia; something for the patient to look at during moments of boredom – and of course, for me too during similar lapses. There was a Hornby OO gauge class 29 BR locomotive, two models of CalMac ships, a couple of miniature Daleks, a *paper mache* vase (lovingly constructed by daughter number three) with 'I love Dad' on it, the rocket that took Tintin to the moon, Thunderbird Three, a number 101 Glasgow trolley-bus (celebrating my own early visits to the dentist, as described earlier) and a small reproduction of an African Star. This array clearly demonstrated to my patients the level of intellectual diversity of their dentist! It certainly brought about some interesting conversations over the years, usually from the guys. The African Star was a World War 2 campaign medal awarded to the Forces personnel who served in Africa; this included my father, who spent four years in Sudan and Egypt with the RAF. My miniature medal was in memory of him and the beady eye of many a patient spotted it hiding behind a dalek. Many asked what it was, or what I had done to earn it. Just one patient – a lady of mature years – recognised the red and yellow colour of its ribbon.

"Why do you have an African Star on your shelf?" I was impressed and she got the full story, of course.

One day, during a break between drills, I looked up and discovered it was gone. I have no idea how it vanished and never saw it again. Perhaps someone had pocketed it, although I wouldn't know why as it was worthless. Fortunately I hadn't put out the real one – which I still have.

Over the years some very hard-faced characters sat in the chair. One chap seemed to have a fresh scar each time he visited us. He would frequently show up as an emergency patient on a Monday morning with yet another loose tooth, stating that he had had a bit of a disagreement with someone. He was a scary character, to be sure; but in the dental chair he was like a lamb – always polite and grateful.

"Thank you Mr Craig."

"See you next Monday, Rocky."

People tended to be pleasant to their dentist – you can imagine why. We once had a minor altercation, however. One morning, just as the surgeries were being set up, a chap crept into my colleague's surgery and walked out with his mini stereo system. Unfortunately for this lad we employed a male dental nurse at the time, who heard a noise and went to investigate. He gave chase to the thief, caught up with him and indulged in a bit of rough justice with the chap's face. Clearly the robber would have to choose a different dentist for his patch-up.

There was another noteworthy event that occurred around this time. We were alerted to it by a young lad who came through the door for his appointment with his eyes almost popping out his head. Apparently there was a lady standing at the street corner just outside our practice repeatedly baring her breasts to passing traffic. Sadly I missed all this, but did wonder what all the horn tooting was for. She was either high on something or thought she was in an Italian layby, but we called the police, who seemed to think it was all quite amusing.

Sometimes younger patients didn't realise that they were to 'check-in' at reception when they arrived for their appointment. I can recall one young lad hiding in a corner of the waiting room for three hours, without anyone wondering who he was and why he was there. Sometimes older patients turned up at the wrong practice. We would then get a phone call from another dental practice informing us that our 1030 patient was sitting in *their* waiting room. One chap even turned up for his scaling at the vet! As I mentioned earlier, I was well capable of presenting myself at the wrong practice too; yes, twice.

Strange coincidences sometimes occur, which the nurses always thought was the work of some unearthly entity. For example we once had just three patients in the waiting room, and they were all called Mrs White. It caused all sorts of confusion when I called: "Mrs White, would you like to come through please?" The three of them became jammed in the door frame. "He meant me!"

Very occasionally we had the luxury of treating a minor celebrity. Neither Susan Sarandon nor Brad Pitt ever enlightened our day, but over the years a few 'well-kent' faces did. I treated a couple of ex-Celtic players but, despite my leaning towards their rivals, I showed complete impartiality during their brief visits to the chair. It was only once they stood up that I let my true inclinations surface. It was all good-spirited of course, and despite one of them breaking my heart at a Scottish Cup Final some years earlier we used to have some great laughs and reminiscences. I also treated a midfield player who had a significant career with Falkirk. I saw his bloodied face late one Saturday night during the football highlights on BBC's *Sportscene*. He wasn't a patient of mine at the time. So imagine my surprise when he turned up at our surgery on the Monday morning with a badly smashed front tooth. I fixed him up, his club paid the bill and he became a regular patient. But why he came to me in the first place I will never know.

My colleague had the pleasure of improving the dental appearance of a well-known Scottish actor, who politely remonstrated that he made his living trying to look unattractive, and that my colleague was trying to undo that.

I also had the pleasure of having a young lady actor on my books. She appeared in annual pantomimes and had several TV screen roles in some well-known Scottish dramas and soaps. I found this very interesting and whenever she came into the surgery I would ask her what she was 'appearing in' lately. On one such occasion, however, I took the opportunity to make a complete fool of myself. This day, she replied to my query by stating that she was appearing in a play at Glasgow's Pavilion Theatre.

"Oh really, how interesting, would I like it? What's it called?"

"It's called *The Vagina Monologues.*"

I'd never heard of it, but without even considering this for the briefest of seconds I found myself asking her, to my horror "so, what's that about then?"

I cannot recall her response as I was too busy trying to hide my blushing face away. I still feel embarrassed when I think of that today. I wanted to phone her later and apologise, but how would I have worded that?

Oh dear, I can give you several examples of other stupid remarks that I trotted out over the years.

"Tell me Mrs Plump when is your baby due?"

"Eh I'm not pregnant, I've just put on a bit of weight and I'm wearing an old curtain that looks like a maternity dress."

Or: "hallo Ms Primm, are you still on the contraceptive pill? And what is it you work at again?"

"I'm a nun."

The four year old attending for the first time, preferring to sit on his grandfather's knee rather than the dental chair.

"That's OK Jimmy, you can sit on Grandad's knee while I look at your teeth."

"Eh, I'm his father, not his pappy!"

And one unforgivable slip, that we were well warned about during our training, but which I still blurted out one day to another wee lad: "your teeth are great, Bobby, now do you want to go into the waiting room and bring your mum in for a chat."

"I don't have a mummy, she's dead." I only made that mistake once. The obvious way around that one is to ask "...and who is with you today Bobby?"

Sometimes one of our patients had their fifteen minutes of fame around the time of their visits to the practice. I spotted one lady appearing on my lunchtime TV screen on a pan-European quiz show called 'Going for Gold'. There she was, doing rather well answering a battery of general knowledge questions. A couple of weeks later she was in the surgery discussing the provision of a crown for a heavily filled and broken back molar. I didn't let on I had seen her screen appearance but during the discussion of her crown I couldn't contain myself any longer.

"So decision time, Mary. Do you want a porcelain crown or are you *going for gold*?"

One type of person that all dentists hate to treat is – you've guessed it – other dentists. We have all treated our fair share of dental colleagues and most of my share was fine. One long-retired dentist was particularly difficult, however, as he just wanted to tell me what to do all the time. I felt like handing him a mirror and a set of instruments and telling him to get on with it. Another ex-dentist - a charming chap - appeared out of the blue one morning wanting an extraction. I was flattered but terrified. As I was just about to extract his molar my endearing colleague opened my surgery door, peered in and said "it's okay Pat, he's holding the right end of the forceps!"

I am of course now in that position; of being the retired dentist who is now a patient, and I feel so sorry for the poor chap in whose capable hands I place myself.

Aside from treating famous patients, there have been a few famous, and infamous, dentists popping up in the annals of history. One of the best known was that well known gambler and gunslinger Doc Holliday, of *Gunfight at the OK Corral* fame.

John Holliday was born in Georgia in 1851 and by the age of twenty-one was a dentist, having obtained his degree from Pennsylvania College. He is infamous for being a gambler, a gunfighter and for suffering from tuberculosis, the disease that eventually killed him at the young age of 36. Moving to Texas for the benefit of his health, Holliday led a somewhat colourful life and befriended the Earp brothers Wyatt, Morgan and Virgil. By the time he moved to Tombstone, Arizona, where Virgil was US marshal, Holliday had given up his dental practice and made his money from gambling. He was made a deputy marshal, under Virgil, and became involved in the well documented shootout at the OK Corral, that little *tete a tete* with the Clanton brothers.

In an earlier chapter I mentioned the use of vulcanite in dentistry. Its invention, and particularly its application to dentures - in the mid 1850s - reduced the costs of denture construction at a time when the prostheses were becoming much in demand. Unfortunately for the dentists of the time, the Goodyear Dental Vulcanite Company realised they were onto a good thing, and wanted a share of the action – or at the very least a fee from every dentist who used vulcanite. This was in the form of an annual licensing fee of $45. This was a not insignificant amount at the time and some dentists rebelled. Goodyear employed his treasurer Josiah Bacon to find the errant dentists and make them pay. One of these was Delaware dentist Samuel Chalfont, who not only refused to pay, but fled westwards across the country. Bacon eventually tracked him to San Francisco where a heated confrontation took place in a hotel. Chalfont shot Bacon dead. He turned himself into the police and eventually served just six years in prison. There was a fair amount of sympathy for him as his victim had been lining his own pockets with some of the licensing fees, so maybe he was a latter day Robin Hood.

No such accolade could be offered for Glennon Engleman, however. He was an American professional hitman who died in prison in 1999 while serving life sentences for a whole upper set of killings. Yes. I am ashamed to say he was a dentist, who found he could make more cash from filling graves than filling teeth.

In modern times few dentists were as infamous as David J. Acer, an American dentist from Ohio who was accused of deliberately infecting six of his patients with the HIV virus. The crucial word here is 'deliberate'. As I mentioned earlier, the chances of picking up an infection at the dentist, apart from the common cold from the guy sneezing next to you in the waiting room, is as close to nil as can be. What Acer is accused of is a heinous crime. Practising in Florida, Acer acquired AIDS and eventually died from it in 1990. It is believed that he deliberately infected some of his patients with the virus, but just how he did it, if he did, and why remains a puzzle.

Dentists have been portrayed on film many times, as you will be aware. My favourite is a short 1932 Mack Sennett film *The Dentist*, starring the inimitable WC Fields. This film was censored for many years, supposedly because it showed the dental profession in a very poor light. Fields' contempt for his patients is quite clear but I feel that the censor was more concerned with the scene where, on trying to extract a tooth from a female patient, he staggers around the room with his patient clinging onto him - her legs wrapped around his waist.

Steve Martin gave another unscrupulous portrayal of a sadistic dentist in the aforementioned 1986 film *Little Shop of Horrors*, and Bob Monkhouse demonstrated the more entrepreneurial side to dentistry in the 1960 and 1961 duo *Dentist in the Chair* and *Dentist on the Job*. Other dentist portrayals include Jennifer Aniston (*Horrible Bosses*) and Ed Helms (*Hangover*).

There are two well-known dentist sequences that make even me cringe however. The first is from the 1992 TV appearance of Rowan Atkinson in *The Trouble with Mr Bean*. The dentist is brilliantly characterised by the perpetually irascible Richard Wilson. It is the sequence where Mr Bean starts to drill his own teeth with a high-speed drill that gives me that hollow feeling in my stomach. The noise of the handpiece and his ardent focus of concentration are disconcertingly realistic, especially when I think about the damage he could be doing.

But the one Mr Nasty whom patients seem to remember and recoil from most was Dr Szell, the Nazi dentist portrayed by Laurence Olivier in John Schlesinger's 1976 film *Marathon Man*. Yes, it is that awful scene where Dustin Hoffman is strapped to the dental chair having his front incisor drilled through to the pulp with Szell uttering those perplexing words "is it safe?" And here I have a terrible admission. In my surgery I had a fairly large hand mirror, which I could hand to patients after completion of some cosmetically pleasing work, so that they could admire their new look – just as they do at the hairdressers. On the back of that mirror I had a photo of Olivier from that scene, drill in hand, poised over the hapless Hoffman. I lost count of the number of times patients would mention that film scene, especially when they were about to have a root- treatment on their front incisor. When they did, and if I thought their nervous state could cope with it, I spun the mirror around. Fortunately nobody ever ran out the door, nor reported me to the General Dental Council, but then, I could usually tell when a patient had a sense of humour. Some of these little moments were hilarious for us all, of course: "tell me Mr Craig, did you ever see that film *Marathon Man* when Dustin Hoffman gets his tooth drilled with no anaesthetic?" Out came the mirror. "Do you mean this one?" On other suitable occasions I didn't need the mirror. I could just glance at my nurse while leaning over a cavity and utter "is it safe?" Fortunately my patients knew me well by this stage in my career.

All these may be entertaining but, as I said at the outset, it would be nice if dentists were one day depicted on the silver screen as the kind, altruistic, philanthropic people that they really are!

As I write this it is three years since I retired. I hung up the mirror and probe after 33 years in practice, a couple of years short of my 60th birthday. I felt I had been doing the same job for all of those years. Dentistry is unusual, in that as one gets older there is no delegation of work – it is still the dentist that performs the operational side of the business. Clearly there are other similar professions – teaching, for example, and medicine. As I reached the end of my career there was a tendency to look over my shoulder at the changes that were coming up on the outside lane. Dentistry is certainly changing, with a shift away from 'family' practices to corporate clinics. The terminology is changing, as in every field, of course. I first noticed it when the term 'personnel' became 'human resources' – a totally ridiculous expression if you ask me, which of course you're not. Maybe it was the embarrassing mess I got into over this subtle realignment of someone who deals with employees. A young lady was sitting in the chair one afternoon and I asked her what she did.

"HR," was her perfunctory reply.

"Hormone Replacement?" I heard myself respond, and immediately regretting it.

Worse was to come. Sitting in the chair, listening to his dentist's choice of music emanating from the speakers behind him, a young lad asked "Cool music, do you use Bluetooth?"

"Oh thank you," I reply, "that's just one of my 112 cassettes. Bluetooth? No we don't do teeth tattoos, but I do tooth-whitening!" Time to retire.

I could wax lyrical about the fantastic voyage or brilliant adventure from student to experienced dentist, but really it was all about a career choice. I could have been that electrical engineer and turned out a different person after all. But that is fate. I have no regrets about my choice of vocation. I didn't set the world on fire, dentally speaking, but I must have influenced a few folk over the years. I felt particularly humbled when two lads I treated over the years eventually became dentists themselves and told me that I had left a mark on them; not a bruise, I hope.

I meet former patients daily, usually in Morrisons, and many ask if I miss it, or if I work part time. I don't miss it but clearly part of my brain does, for I dream about working on teeth regularly. There is always an impediment in the dream: I am 'fixing' teeth, but know I am doing so illegally, although the receptionist keeps telling me no one will ever find out.

Working part time was not an option for me, as there are insurances, annual registrations, medical sickness cover which all add up and make it unviable.

It was a real honour to be a dentist. Having the trust of your patients and being able to help them defined the kind of person I ultimately became, from the green, *Job Creation Scheme* graduate, to the (hopefully) mature and wiser practice owner. I didn't get things right all the time – I will have let some people down over all these years, but I tried my best and was always honest with the people whom I had the privilege of caring for. The greatest asset a new graduate dentist possesses is their education. The greatest asset the mature dentist has is experience – knowing how to adapt to ongoing situations daily, and understanding one's own limitations and knowing that you can still get caught out by that molar that doesn't really want to part from its host.

Now I have a daughter who is a dentist, and grandchildren who may enter the profession one day. My mother was amazed when I told her at the age of fifteen that I was going to be a dentist. I actually amazed myself when I finally graduated as one. For those considering the profession as a career – embrace it! Be honest to yourself and your patients, and work hard. A whole diverse assortment of rewards is just around the corner.

Oh, I almost forgot – my *Rolling Stones* story! Just ask any of my patients, they'll tell you it.

ACKNOWLEDGEMENTS

Many thanks go to my former colleague, Alan Caplan, for approving my account of our professional partnership, which extended to over 25 years. I also thank my former dental nurses who gave me the nod to go ahead and chronical most of their funny ways. Some of their stories had to be left out, and all their names have been changed - but you all know who you are.

Further gratitude is due to Donny McIvor who proof-read the manuscript and even came with me to the dentist back in 1974 to offer reassurance.

The library at Glasgow Dental Hospital were very helpful to me and, of course, I thank Glasgow University for educating me on how to be a professional and helping set me up for life. Graeme Jamieson gave me my first job and he and David Lawson helped me tremendously in the early part of my career. Thanks chaps.

Thanks are due to the Oral Health Foundation Dental Helpline for their help and for the support they give to patients regarding their dental treatment.

Cover photograph reproduced courtesy of Lewis Segal.

Thanks to Fiona Louise Craig for her line drawings of the canine and molar, and to Gemma at United Dental Care for her help.

Finally, thank you patients. I couldn't have done it without you and I loved you all – well, most of you!